Readings on Diarrhoea

Student manual

World Health Organization
Geneva
1992

WHO Library Cataloguing in Publication Data

Readings on diarrhoea: student manual.

1. Diarrhea, Infantile — programmed instruction

ISBN 92 4 154444 9 (NLM Classification: WS 18)

Typeset in India
Printed in Belgium
91/8972–Macmillan/Ceuterick–9000

Contents

Preface

This manual is intended for medical students, especially during their clinical training in paediatrics. It will also be useful for physicians participating in training courses on the management of diarrhoea in children. The materials in this book are compatible with other WHO publications on the management and prevention of diarrhoea. The units that concern the management of children with diarrhoea are based on the WHO treatment chart "Management of the Patient with Diarrhoea" (1992), portions of which are reproduced at appropriate places in this text.

This book may be used as a source of practical information and as a manual of guidelines for treating patients with diarrhoea. It will be more effective, however, if used in combination with organized teaching activities on diarrhoeal diseases, such as lectures, discussions, demonstrations, and supervised practice in treating cases. Readers are urged to check their understanding of the material by answering the questions that follow each unit. A companion book *References on diarrhoea* contains related background articles that summarize current research and provide additional information on most topics covered in this text. This is available[1] to medical school libraries and other institutions conducting training in diarrhoea case management. An *Instructor's manual* is also available,[1] which provides guidance for medical faculty and other teachers about how the material in each unit of the text may be most effectively taught.

[1]Available on request from the Division of Diarrhoeal and Acute Respiratory Disease Control, World Health Organization, 1211 Geneva 27, Switzerland.

Acknowledgements

This publication is based on a manual prepared by Dr R. S. Northrup of the Technology for Primary Health Care Project (PRITECH), under contract from WHO. It has been reviewed by Dr D. Bratt, Department of Paediatrics, University of the West Indies, Trinidad and Tobago; Dr W. A. M. Cutting, Department of Child Health, University of Edinburgh, Edinburgh, Scotland; Dr L. Gothefors, Department of Paediatrics, University of Umea, Umea, Sweden; Dr D. Habte, International Centre for Diarrhoeal Diseases Research, Dhaka, Bangladesh; and Dr M. Khan, The Children's Hospital, Pakistan Institute of Medical Sciences, Karachi, Pakistan.

UNIT 1

The epidemiology and etiology of diarrhoea

Introduction

Diarrhoea is a leading cause of illness and death among children in developing countries, where an estimated 1.3 thousand million episodes and 3.2 million deaths occur each year in those under five years of age. Overall, these children experience an average of 3.3 episodes of diarrhoea per year, but in some areas the average exceeds nine episodes per year. Where episodes are frequent, young children may spend more than 15% of their days with diarrhoea (Fig. 1.1). About 80% of deaths due to diarrhoea occur in the first 2 years of life. The main cause of death from acute diarrhoea is dehydration, which results from the loss of fluid and electrolytes in diarrhoeal stools. Other important causes of death are dysentery, malnutrition and serious infections, such as pneumonia.

Diarrhoea is an important cause of malnutrition. This is because patients with diarrhoea eat less and their ability to absorb nutrients is reduced; moreover, their nutrient requirements are increased as a result of the infection. Each episode of diarrhoea contributes to malnutrition; when episodes are prolonged, their impact on growth is increased.

Diarrhoeal disease also represents an economic burden for the developing countries. In many countries, more than one-third of hospital beds for children are occupied by patients with diarrhoea. These patients are often treated with expensive intravenous fluids and ineffective drugs. Although diarrhoeal disease is usually less harmful to adults than to children, it can also affect a country's economy by reducing the health of its workforce.

Fig. 1.1 **Prevalence of diarrhoea in different developing countries**

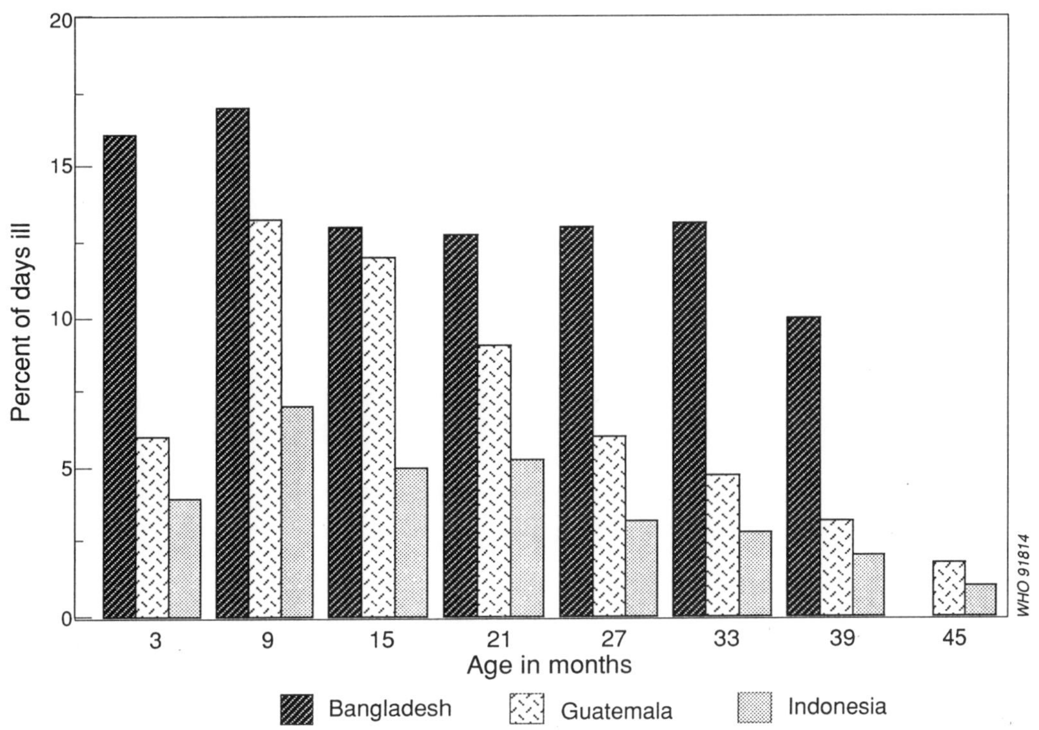

Source: Rohde, J. & Northrup, R.S. Diarrhoea is a nutritional disease. In: Ladislaus-Sanei, L. & Scully, P.E., ed. *ICORT II Proceedings—Second International Conference on Oral Rehydration Therapy, Washington, DC, 10–13 December 1985.* Washington, DC, Agency for International Development, 1986, pp. 30–41.

Fortunately, simple and effective treatment measures are available that can markedly reduce the number of deaths caused by diarrhoea, make admission to hospital unnecessary in most cases, and prevent the adverse effect of diarrhoea on nutritional status. Practical preventive measures can also be taken that substantially reduce the incidence and severity of diarrhoeal episodes. This unit provides information on the epidemiology and etiology of diarrhoea that is essential for understanding the principles of treatment and prevention.

Types of diarrhoea

Diarrhoea is usually defined in epidemiological studies as the passage of three or more loose or watery stools in a 24-hour period, a loose stool being one that would take the shape of a container. However, mothers may use a variety of terms to describe diarrhoea, depending, for example, upon whether the stool is loose, watery, bloody or mucoid, or there is vomiting. It is important to be familiar with these terms when asking whether a child has diarrhoea. Infants who are exclusively breast-fed normally pass several soft or semi-liquid stools each day; for them, it is practical to define diarrhoea as an increase in stool frequency or liquidity that is considered abnormal by the mother.

Three clinical syndromes of diarrhoea have been defined, each reflecting a different pathogenesis and requiring different approaches to treatment. These are described briefly below and considered in detail in Units 3–6.

Acute watery diarrhoea

This term refers to diarrhoea that begins acutely, lasts less than 14 days (most episodes last less than 7 days), and involves the passage of frequent loose or watery stools without visible blood. Vomiting may occur and fever may be present. Acute watery diarrhoea causes dehydration; when food intake is reduced, it also contributes to malnutrition. When death occurs, it is usually due to acute dehydration. The most important causes of acute watery diarrhoea in young children in developing countries are rotavirus, enterotoxigenic *Escherichia coli*, *Shigella*, *Campylobacter jejuni*, and *Cryptosporidium*. In some areas, *Vibrio cholerae* O1, *Salmonella* and enteropathogenic *E. coli* are also important.

Dysentery

This is diarrhoea with visible blood in the faeces. Important effects of dysentery include anorexia, rapid weight loss, and damage to the intestinal mucosa by the invasive bacteria. A number of other complications may also occur. The main cause of acute dysentery is *Shigella*; other causes are *Campylobacter jejuni* and, infrequently, enteroinvasive *E. coli* or *Salmonella*. *Entamoeba histolytica* can cause serious dysentery in young adults but is rarely a cause of dysentery in young children.

Persistent diarrhoea

This is diarrhoea that begins acutely but is of unusually long duration (at least 14 days). The episode may begin either as watery diarrhoea or as dysentery. Marked weight loss is frequent. Diarrhoeal stool volume may also be great, with a risk of dehydration. There is no single microbial cause for persistent diarrhoea; entero-aggregative *E. coli*, *Shigella* and *Cryptosporidium* may play a greater role than other agents. Persistent diarrhoea should not be confused with chronic diarrhoea, which is recurrent or long-lasting diarrhoea due to noninfectious causes, such as sensitivity to gluten or inherited metabolic disorders.

Epidemiology

Transmission of agents that cause diarrhoea

The infectious agents that cause diarrhoea are usually spread by the faecal–oral route, which includes the ingestion of faecally contaminated water or food, and direct contact with infected faeces.

A number of specific behaviours promote the transmission of enteric pathogens and thus increase the risk of diarrhoea. These include:

- *Failing to breast-feed exclusively for the first 4–6 months of life.* The risk of developing severe diarrhoea is many times greater in infants who are not breast-fed than in those who are exclusively breast-fed; the risk of death from diarrhoea is also substantially greater.

- *Using infant feeding bottles.* These easily become contaminated with faecal bacteria and are difficult to clean. When milk is added to an unclean bottle it becomes contaminated; if it is not consumed immediately, bacterial growth occurs.

- *Storing cooked food at room temperature.* When food is cooked and then saved to be used later, it may easily be contaminated, for example, by contact with contaminated surfaces or containers. If food is kept for several hours at room temperature, bacteria in it can multiply many times.

- *Using drinking-water contaminated with faecal bacteria.* Water may be contaminated at its source or during storage in the home. Contamination in the home may occur when the storage container is not covered, or when a contaminated hand comes into contact with the water while collecting it from the container.

- *Failing to wash hands after defecation, after disposing of faeces or before handling food.*

- *Failing to dispose of faeces (including infant faeces) hygienically.* It is often believed that infant faeces are harmless, whereas they may actually contain large numbers of infectious viruses or bacteria; animal faeces can also transmit enteric infections to humans.

Host factors that increase susceptibility to diarrhoea

Several host factors are associated with increased incidence, severity, or duration of diarrhoea. They include:

- *Failing to breast-feed until at least 2 years of age.* Breast milk contains antibodies that protect against certain types of diarrhoeal disease, such as shigellosis and cholera.

- *Malnutrition.* The severity, duration, and risk of death from diarrhoea are increased in malnourished children, especially those with severe malnutrition.

- *Measles.* Diarrhoea and dysentery are more frequent or severe in children with measles or who have had measles in the previous 4 weeks. This presumably results from immunological impairment caused by measles.

- *Immunodeficiency or immunosuppression.* This may be temporary, e.g. after certain viral infections (e.g. measles), or it may be prolonged, as in people with acquired immunodeficiency syndrome (AIDS). When immunosuppression is severe, diarrhoea can be caused by unusual pathogens and may also be prolonged.

Age

Most diarrhoeal episodes occur during the first 2 years of life. Incidence is highest in the age group 6–11 months, when weaning often occurs (Fig. 1.2). This pattern reflects the combined effects of declining levels of maternally acquired antibodies, the lack of active immunity in the infant, the introduction of food that may be contaminated with faecal bacteria, and direct contact with human or animal faeces when the infant starts to crawl. Most enteric pathogens stimulate at least partial immunity against repeated infection or illness, which helps to explain the declining incidence of disease in older children and adults.

Fig. 1.2 **Estimated median diarrhoeal morbidity rates for children under 5 years of age, by age group**

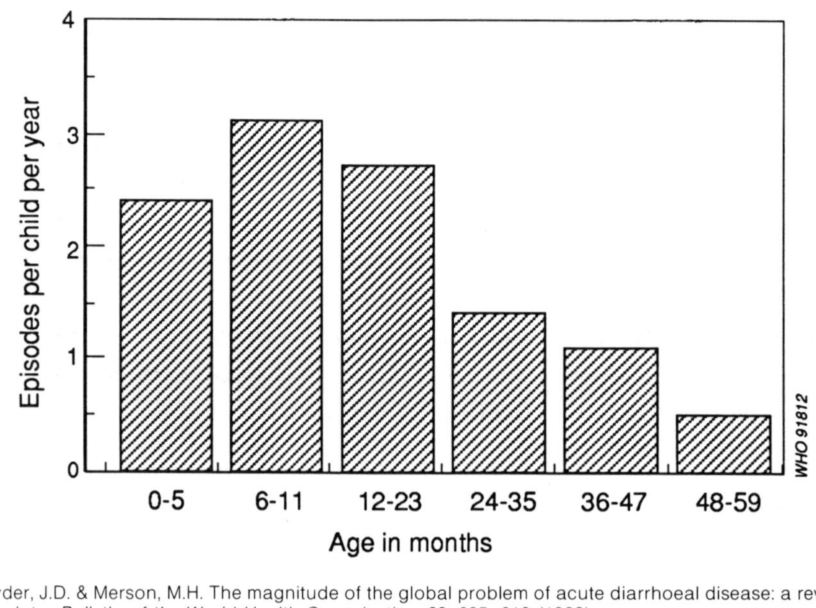

Source: Snyder, J.D. & Merson, M.H. The magnitude of the global problem of acute diarrhoeal disease: a review of active surveillance data. *Bulletin of the World Health Organization*, **60**: 605–613 (1982).

Seasonality

Distinct seasonal patterns of diarrhoea occur in many geographical areas. In temperate climates, bacterial diarrhoeas occur more frequently during the warm season, whereas viral diarrhoeas, particularly diarrhoea caused by rotavirus, peak during the winter. In tropical areas, rotavirus diarrhoea occurs throughout the year, increasing in frequency during the drier, cool months, whereas bacterial diarrhoeas peak during the warmer, rainy season. The incidence of persistent diarrhoea follows the same seasonal pattern as that of acute watery diarrhoea.

Asymptomatic infections

Most enteric infections are asymptomatic, and the proportion that is asymptomatic increases beyond 2 years of age owing to the development of active immunity. During asymptomatic infections, which may last for several days or weeks, stools contain infectious viruses, bacteria, or protozoal cysts. People with asymptomatic infections play an important role in the spread of many enteric pathogens, especially as they are unaware of their infection, take no special hygienic precautions and move normally from place to place.

Epidemics

Two enteric pathogens, *Vibrio cholerae* O1 and *Shigella dysenteriae* type 1, cause major epidemics in which morbidity and mortality in all age groups may be high. Since 1961, cholera caused by the eltor biotype of *V. cholerae* O1 has spread to countries in Africa, Latin America, Asia, and the Eastern Mediterranean, and to some areas in North America and Europe. During the same period, *S. dysenteriae* type 1 has been responsible for large epidemics of severe dysentery in Central America, and more recently in Central Africa and southern Asia.

Etiology

General considerations

Until a few years ago, pathogenic organisms could be identified in the faeces of only about 25% of patients with acute diarrhoea. Today, using new techniques, experienced laboratory technicians can identify pathogens in about 75% of cases seen at a treatment facility and up to 50% of milder cases detected in the community.

The organisms most frequently associated with diarrhoea in young children in developing countries are shown in Table 1.1. Several of these pathogens are important causes of acute diarrhoea in all developing countries. They are:

- rotavirus
- enterotoxigenic *Escherichia coli*
- *Shigella*
- *Campylobacter jejuni*
- *Cryptosporidium*.

Table 1.1 **Pathogens frequently identified in children with acute diarrhoea seen at treatment centres in developing countries**

	Pathogen	Percentage of cases	Recommended antimicrobial based on clinical signs[a]
Viruses	Rotavirus	15–25	None
Bacteria	Enterotoxigenic *Escherichia coli*	10–20	None
	Shigella	5–15	Trimethoprim–sulfamethoxazole, nalidixic acid
	Campylobacter jejuni	10–15	None
	Vibrio cholerae O1	5–10[b]	Tetracycline[c]
	Salmonella (non-typhoid)	1–5	None
	Enteropathogenic *Escherichia coli*	1–5	None
Protozoa	*Cryptosporidium*	5–15	None
No pathogen found		20–30	None

[a] For sensitive strains.
[b] In endemic areas; may be higher during epidemics.
[c] Also effective are furazolidone, trimethoprim–sulfamethoxazole, erythromycin and chloramphenicol.

Others may be of local importance; these include *V. cholerae* O1 (in endemic areas and during epidemics), non-typhoid *Salmonella* (in areas where commercially processed foods are widely used), and enteropathogenic *E. coli* (in infants in hospitals). Mixed infections involving two or more enteropathogens occur in 5–20% of cases seen at health facilities.

A number of other pathogens are not shown in Table 1.1. In general, their role in the etiology of acute diarrhoea in children in developing countries is either minimal or not yet well defined. They include:

- viruses: Norwalk agent, enteric adenoviruses;
- bacteria: *Aeromonas hydrophila*, enteroaggregative *Escherichia coli*, enteroinvasive *E. coli*, enterohaemorrhagic *E. coli*, *Plesiomonas shigelloides*, *Vibrio cholerae* non-O1, *V. parahaemolyticus*, *Yersinia enterocolitica*;
- protozoa: *Giardia lamblia, Entamoeba histolytica, Isospora belli.*

Enteric pathogens can also be found in about 30% of healthy children under 3 years of age, making it difficult to know whether a pathogen isolated from a child with diarrhoea is actually the cause of that child's illness. This is especially true for *Giardia lamblia*, cysts of which are found nearly as often in healthy children as in those with diarrhoea; it is also true for enteropathogenic *E. coli* or *C. jejuni* isolated from children older than 1 year. On the other hand, *Shigella* and rotavirus are rarely identified in healthy children; their presence in a child with diarrhoea is strong evidence that they are causing the illness.

Table 1.1 shows that antimicrobial agents are recommended only when infections with *Shigella* or *V. cholerae* O1 are suspected on the basis of clinical signs. For all other agents, and thus for the *majority* of acute diarrhoeal episodes in young children, antimicrobials are either ineffective (e.g. rotavirus) or the appropriate antimicrobial can only be selected after the agent has been identified by stool culture (e.g. enterotoxigenic *E. coli*). For some agents (e.g. *Salmonella*), the use of an antimicrobial can actually prolong the intestinal infection. *For all of these reasons, antimicrobials should not be given "blindly" or routinely to patients with diarrhoea.* The few instances in which antimicrobials should be used are considered further in Units 5 and 6.

Pathogenetic mechanisms

Microbial agents cause diarrhoea by a number of mechanisms, several of which are considered below.

Viruses

- Viruses, such as rotavirus, replicate within the villous epithelium of the small bowel, causing patchy epithelial cell destruction and villous shortening. The loss of normally absorptive villous cells and their temporary replacement by immature, secretory, crypt-like cells causes the intestine to secrete water and electrolytes. Villous damage may also be associated with the loss of disaccharidase enzymes, leading to reduced absorption of dietary disaccharides, especially lactose. Recovery occurs when the villi regenerate and the villous epithelium matures.

Bacteria

- *Mucosal adhesion.* Bacteria that multiply within the small intestine must first adhere to the mucosa to avoid being swept away. Adhesion is through superficial hair-like antigens, termed pili or fimbriae, that bind to receptors on the intestinal surface; this occurs, for example, with enterotoxigenic *E. coli* and *V. cholerae* O1. In some instances, mucosal adherence is associated with changes in the gut epithelium that may reduce its absorptive capacity or cause fluid secretion (e.g. in infection with enteropathogenic or enteroaggregative *E. coli*).

- *Toxins that cause secretion.* Enterotoxigenic *E. coli*, *V. cholerae* O1 and some other bacteria produce toxins that alter epithelial cell function. These toxins reduce the absorption of sodium by the villi and may increase the secretion of chloride in the crypts, causing secretion of water and electrolytes (see Unit 2). Recovery occurs when the affected cells are replaced by healthy ones after 2–4 days.

- *Mucosal invasion. Shigella*, *C. jejuni*, enteroinvasive *E. coli* and *Salmonella* can cause bloody diarrhoea by invading and destroying mucosal epithelial cells. This occurs mostly in the colon and the distal part of the ileum. Invasion may be followed by the formation of microabscesses and superficial ulcers; hence the presence of red and white blood cells, or visible blood, in the stool. Toxins produced by these organisms cause tissue damage and possibly also mucosal secretion of water and electrolytes.

Protozoa

- *Mucosal adhesion. G. lamblia* and *Cryptosporidium* adhere to the small bowel epithelium and cause shortening of the villi, which may be how they cause diarrhoea.

- *Mucosal invasion. E. histolytica* causes diarrhoea by invading epithelial cells in the colon (or ileum) and causing microabscesses and ulcers. This only happens, however, when the infecting strain of *E. histolytica* is virulent. In about 90% of human infections the strains are nonvirulent; in such cases there is no mucosal invasion and no symptoms occur, although amoebic cysts and trophozoites may be present in the faeces.

Important enteropathogens

Rotavirus

Rotavirus is the most important cause of severe, life-threatening diarrhoea in children under 2 years of age worldwide. There are four serotypes of human rotavirus; infection with one serotype causes a high level of immunity to that serotype, and partial protection against the other serotypes. Nearly all children are infected at least once before the age of 2 years, and repeat infections are common. Usually only the first rotavirus infection causes significant illness. About one-third of children under 2 years of age experience an episode of diarrhoea due to rotavirus. Rotavirus is probably spread by person-to-person transmission.

Enterotoxigenic *Escherichia coli* (ETEC)

Enterotoxigenic *E. coli* (ETEC) is an important cause of acute watery diarrhoea in adults and children in developing countries. ETEC does not invade the bowel mucosa and the diarrhoea it causes is mediated by toxins. There are two ETEC toxins, heat-labile (LT) and heat-stable (ST). Some strains produce only one type of toxin, some both. The LT toxin is closely related to cholera toxin. ETEC is spread mostly by means of contaminated food and water.

Shigella

Shigella is the most important cause of dysentery, being found in about 60% of all episodes, and in nearly all severe episodes; watery diarrhoea may also occur. There are four serogroups: *S. sonnei, S. boydii, S. flexneri* and *S. dysenteriae.*

S. flexneri is the most common serogroup in developing countries, but *S. dysenteriae* type 1, which occurs in regional epidemics, causes the most severe disease. Tissue destruction and possibly watery diarrhoea are caused in part by the extremely potent Shiga toxin, produced in relatively large amounts by *S. dysenteriae* type 1. *Shigella* are spread mostly by person-to-person transmission. Antimicrobials to which *Shigella* are sensitive provide effective treatment, but antimicrobial resistance is common. Resistance to multiple antimicrobials may occur, especially among *S. dysenteriae* type 1. The most useful antimicrobials are trimethoprim–sulfamethoxazole and nalidixic acid; ampicillin is effective in some areas.

Campylobacter jejuni

In developing countries, *C. jejuni* causes disease mostly in infants. *C. jejuni* also infects animals, especially chickens and dogs, and is spread by contact with their faeces or consumption of contaminated food, milk, or water. *C. jejuni* can cause watery diarrhoea (two-thirds of cases) or dysentery (one-third of cases). Fever may be present. Episodes are not usually severe and last 2–5 days. Although erythromycin shortens the illness if given soon after the symptoms start, it is not recommended because cases caused by *C. jejuni* cannot be distinguished clinically from those due to other agents; erythromycin is ineffective if therapy is delayed until the diagnosis is confirmed by a laboratory.

Vibrio cholerae O1

V. cholerae O1, the cause of cholera, has two biotypes (classical and eltor) and two serotypes (Ogawa and Inaba). *V. cholerae* O1 is non-invasive, diarrhoea being mediated by cholera toxin which causes a profuse secretion of water and electrolytes in the small bowel. Diarrhoea may be severe, leading to dehydration, collapse and death within a few hours if the lost fluids and salts are not replaced. In endemic areas, cholera occurs mostly in children, adults having substantial immunity from previous infections. In nonendemic areas, epidemics cause disease with equal frequency in adults and children. Antimicrobials can shorten the duration of the illness and thus simplify case management. Tetracycline (or doxycycline) is most widely used, but resistance has been observed in some areas; in this event, other antimicrobials such as furazolidone, trimethoprim–sulfamethoxazole, erythromycin, or chloramphenicol are usually effective.

Salmonella

Most non-typhoid salmonella infections can be traced to infected animals or contaminated animal products. *Salmonella* are an unusual cause of diarrhoea in most developing countries, but may be important in communities where commercially processed foods are widely used. Diarrhoea is usually watery, but dysentery may occur. Antimicrobials are not effective, and may delay the clearance of *Salmonella* from the intestinal tract.

Cryptosporidium

This is a coccidian parasite that causes diarrhoea in infants, immunodeficient patients, and a variety of domestic animals. In developing countries infection is frequent, and most episodes of illness occur in the first year of life. Thereafter, infections are usually asymptomatic. Diarrhoea is usually neither severe nor prolonged, except in immunodeficient patients, such as those with severe malnutrition or AIDS. In such individuals, *Cryptosporidium* is an important cause of persistent diarrhoea with wasting.

Implications for treatment and prevention of diarrhoea

Treatment of diarrhoea

Routine determination of the etiology of diarrhoea in a laboratory is not practical, and the clinical aspects of the illness do not permit a specific etiological diagnosis to be made with confidence. The treatment of patients with diarrhoea must therefore be based on the major features of the disease and an understanding of the underlying pathogenetic mechanisms. The main principles of treatment are as follows:

- Watery diarrhoea requires replacement of fluids and electrolytes — irrespective of its etiology.

- Feeding should be continued during all types of diarrhoea to the greatest extent possible, and should be increased during convalescence so as to avoid any adverse effect on nutritional status.

- Antimicrobials and antiparasitic agents should not be used routinely; most episodes, including severe diarrhoea and diarrhoea with fever, do not benefit from such treatment. The exceptions are:

  — dysentery, which should be treated with an antimicrobial effective for *Shigella*; the few patients who do not respond to this treatment should be studied further or treated for possible amoebiasis:
  — suspected cholera with severe dehydration;
  — persistent diarrhoea, when trophozoites or cysts of *Giardia* or trophozoites of *E. histolytica* are seen in faeces or intestinal fluid, or when pathogenic enteric bacteria are identified by stool culture.

The treatment of patients with acute watery diarrhoea, dysentery, and persistent diarrhoea is considered in detail in Units 4–7.

Prevention of diarrhoea

Measures that interrupt the transmission of pathogens

The various infectious agents that cause diarrhoea are all transmitted by common faecal–oral pathways, such as contaminated water, food, and hands. Measures taken to interrupt the transmission of the causative agents should focus on these pathways. Important measures of proven efficacy include:

- giving only breast milk for the first 4–6 months of life;
- avoiding the use of infant feeding bottles;
- improving practices related to the preparation and storage of weaning foods (to minimize microbial contamination and growth);
- using clean water for drinking;
- washing hands (after defecation or disposing of faeces, and before preparing food or eating);
- safely disposing of faeces, including those of infants.

Measures that strengthen host defences

A number of risk factors for frequent or severe diarrhoea reflect impaired host defences. Measures that can be taken to improve host defences and thus diminish the risk of diarrhoea include:

- continuing to breast-feed for at least the first 2 years of life;
- improving nutritional status (by improving the nutritional value of weaning foods and giving children more food);
- immunizing against measles.

Measures to prevent diarrhoea are considered in greater detail in Unit 8.

Exercises

1. For which of the following reasons is diarrhoea in young children an important public health problem? (There may be more than one correct answer.)

   A. It places a heavy burden on health facilities and resources.
   B. It is a major cause of mortality in young children.
   C. It contributes to malnutrition in young children.
   D. It accounts for a large proportion of the days of illness in young children.

2. Mohan is 9 months old and was healthy until he developed diarrhoea 3 weeks ago. The episode began with stools that were loose and sometimes watery. Mohan has vomited several times in the past week. His mother says that he is not eating as much as usual and seems to have lost weight. He was weaned from breast milk to cow's milk 6 weeks ago. What type of diarrhoea does Mohan have?

   A. Acute diarrhoea.
   B. Acute dysentery.
   C. Chronic diarrhoea.
   D. Allergic diarrhoea.
   E. Persistent diarrhoea.

3. List the 5 most important causes of acute diarrhoea among children in developing countries (including viral, bacterial, and protozoal agents).
   A. ____________________
   B. ____________________
   C. ____________________
   D. ____________________
   E. ____________________

4. In what proportion of cases can the etiology of acute watery diarrhoea be *correctly* determined on the basis of the clinical features of the illness?

   A. 0%.
   B. 10%.
   C. 25%.
   D. 40%.
   E. 75%.

5. In which of the following situations is it correct to give an antimicrobial to a child with diarrhoea? (There may be more than one correct answer.)

   A. The child has had bloody diarrhoea with fever for 2 days.
   B. The child has watery diarrhoea and the family keeps chickens.
   C. The child has had watery diarrhoea with fever for 2 days.
   D. The child has severe dehydration from acute watery diarrhoea and cases of cholera have recently been confirmed in the area.
   E. The child has had diarrhoea for 12 days and shows signs of dehydration and weight loss.

6. Which of the following agents are important causes of acute diarrhoea or dysentery in young children in most developing countries? (There may be more than one correct answer.)

   A. *Entamoeba histolytica.*
   B. *Yersinia enterocolitica.*
   C. Enterohaemorrhagic *Escherichia coli.*
   D. Enterotoxigenic *Escherichia coli.*
   E. *Plesiomonas shigelloides.*

7. Which of the following factors can reduce the incidence or severity of diarrhoea in young children? (There may be more than one correct answer.)

   A. Washing hands after defecation and before preparing food.
   B. Bathing the child frequently.
   C. Exclusive breast-feeding for the first 4–6 months of life.
   D. Immunizing against diphtheria, pertussis and tetanus (DPT).
   E. Immunizing against measles.

UNIT 2

Pathophysiology of watery diarrhoea: dehydration and rehydration

Intestinal physiology

Watery diarrhoea is caused by a disturbance in the mechanism of transport of water and electrolytes in the small intestine. Intestinal transport mechanisms are also the basis for the management of diarrhoea, through oral rehydration therapy and feeding. It is therefore important to understand some of the normal mechanisms of intestinal transport and how they are altered during diarrhoea.

Normal intestinal fluid balance

Normally, absorption and secretion of water and electrolytes occur throughout the intestine. For example, a healthy adult takes in about 2 litres of fluid each day. Saliva and secretions from the stomach, pancreas, and liver add about 7 litres, making a total of about 9 litres of fluid that enter the small intestine every day. There, water and electrolytes are simultaneously absorbed by the villi and secreted by the crypts of the bowel epithelium. This causes a two-directional flow of water and electrolytes between the intestinal lumen and the blood. Since fluid absorption is normally greater than fluid secretion, the *net* result is fluid absorption (see Fig. 2.1, part 1).

Usually, more than 90% of the fluid entering the small intestine is absorbed, so that about 1 litre reaches the large intestine. There, further absorption occurs, only 100 to 200 millilitres of water being excreted each day in formed stools. Any change in the two-directional flow of water and electrolytes in the small intestine (i.e. increased secretion, decreased absorption, or both) results in either reduced net absorption or actual net secretion and causes an increased volume of fluid to enter the large intestine. When this volume exceeds the limited absorptive capacity of the large intestine, diarrhoea occurs.

Intestinal absorption of water and electrolytes

Absorption of water from the small intestine is caused by osmotic gradients that are created when solutes (particularly sodium) are actively absorbed from the bowel lumen by the villous epithelial cells. There are several mechanisms whereby sodium is absorbed in the small intestine (see Fig. 2.2, part 1). To enter the epithelial cells, sodium is linked to the absorption of chloride ion (example A), or absorbed directly as sodium ion (example B), or exchanged for hydrogen ion (example C), or linked to the absorption of organic substances such as glucose or certain amino acids (example D). The addition of glucose to an electrolyte solution can increase sodium absorption in the small intestine as much as threefold.

After being absorbed, sodium is transported out of the epithelial cells by an ion pump referred to as $Na^{+}K^{+}$ATPase. This transfers sodium into the extracellular fluid (ECF), elevating its osmolality and causing water and other electrolytes to flow passively from the small bowel lumen through intercellular channels and into the ECF (see Fig. 2.2, part 1). This process maintains an osmotic balance between fluid in the bowel lumen and the ECF.

Intestinal secretion of water and electrolytes

Secretion of water and electrolytes normally occurs in the crypts of the small bowel epithelium, where sodium chloride is transported from the ECF into the epithelial cell

Fig. 2.1 **Absorption and secretion of electrolytes and water by intestinal epithelium**

1. Normal small intestine

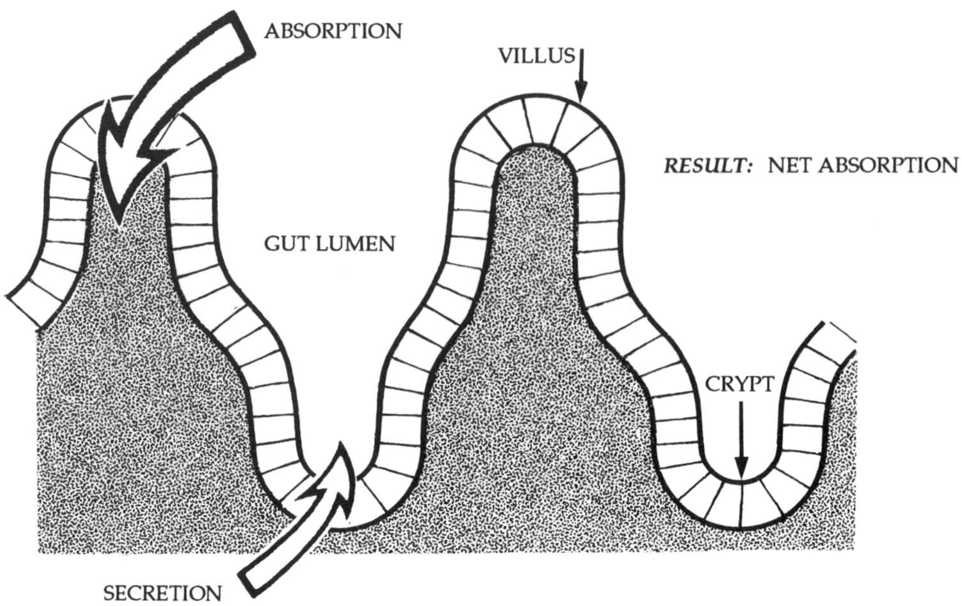

2. Secretory diarrhoea

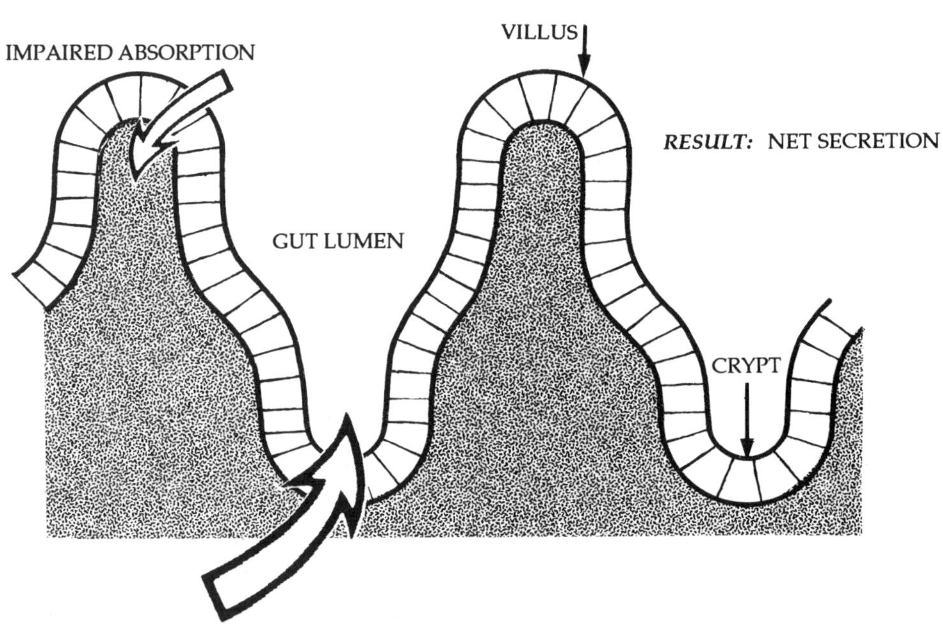

WHO 89961

across its basolateral membrane (see Fig. 2.2, part 2). The sodium is then pumped back into the ECF by Na^+K^+ATPase. At the same time, secretory stimuli cause chloride ions to pass through the luminal membrane of the crypt cells, into the bowel lumen. This creates an osmotic gradient that causes water and other electrolytes to flow passively from the ECF into the bowel lumen through the intercellular channels.

Fig. 2.2 **Mechanisms of absorption and secretion of electrolytes and water in the small bowel epithelium**

1. Sodium absorption in the villous epithelium

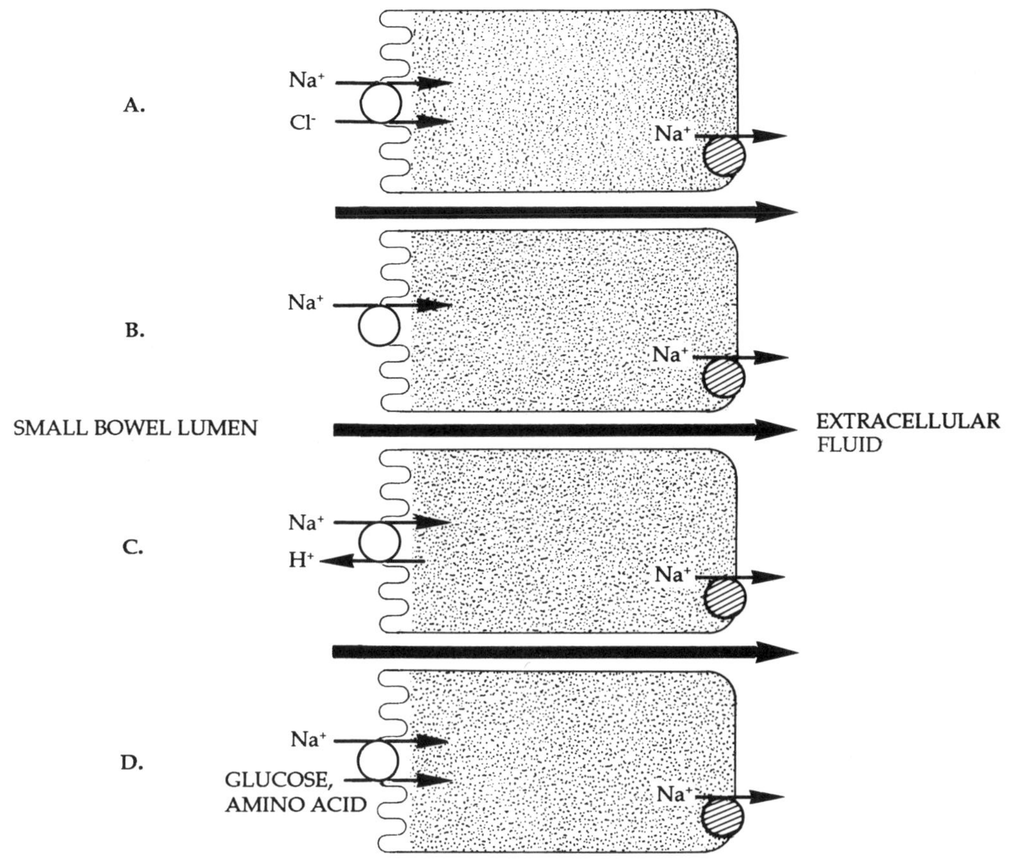

2. Chloride secretion in the crypt epithelium

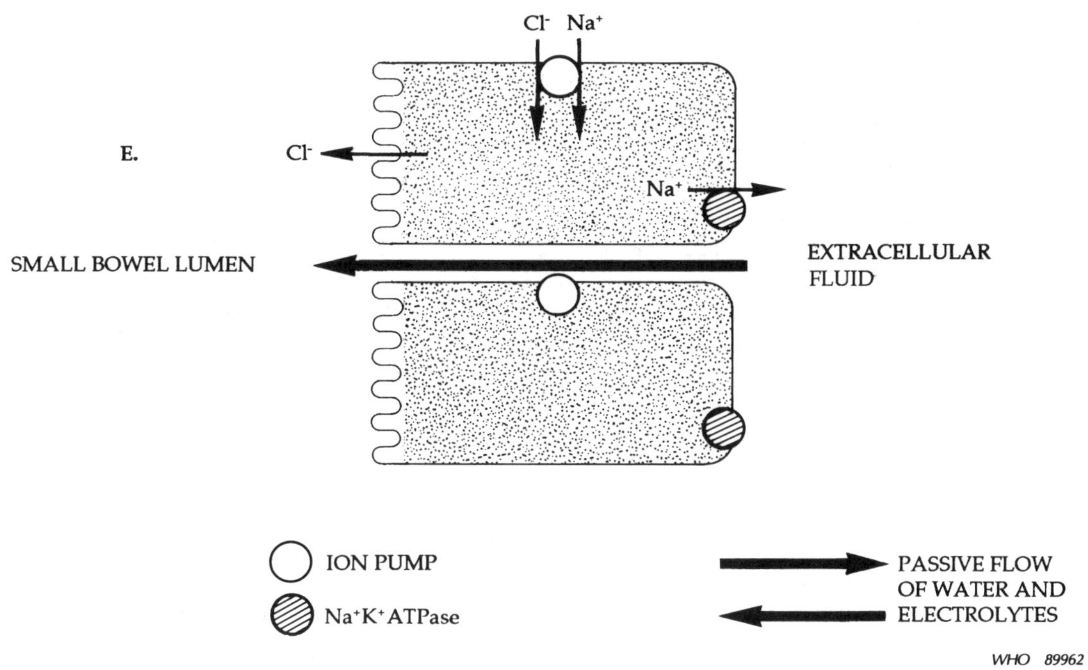

Mechanisms of watery diarrhoea

There are two principal mechanisms by which watery diarrhoea occurs: (i) secretion, and (ii) osmotic action. Intestinal infections can cause diarrhoea by both mechanisms, secretory diarrhoea being more common, and both may occur in a single individual.

Secretory diarrhoea

Secretory diarrhoea is caused by the abnormal secretion of water and electrolytes into the small bowel. This occurs when the absorption of sodium by the villi is impaired while the secretion of chloride in the crypt cells continues or is increased (see Fig. 2.1, part 2). The net result is fluid secretion, which leads to the loss of water and salts from the body as watery stools; this causes dehydration. In infectious diarrhoea, these changes may result from the action on the bowel mucosa of bacterial toxins, such as those of *Escherichia coli* and *Vibrio cholerae* O1,or of viruses, such as rotavirus; other mechanisms may also be important.

Osmotic diarrhoea

The small bowel mucosa is a porous epithelium, across which water and electrolytes move rapidly to maintain osmotic balance between the bowel contents and the ECF. Under these conditions, diarrhoea can occur when a poorly absorbed, osmotically active substance is ingested. If the substance is taken as an *isotonic* solution, the water and solute will simply pass through the gut unabsorbed, causing diarrhoea (see Fig. 2.3, A). Purgatives, such as magnesium sulfate, work by this principle. The same

Fig. 2.3 **Mechanisms of osmotic diarrhoea**

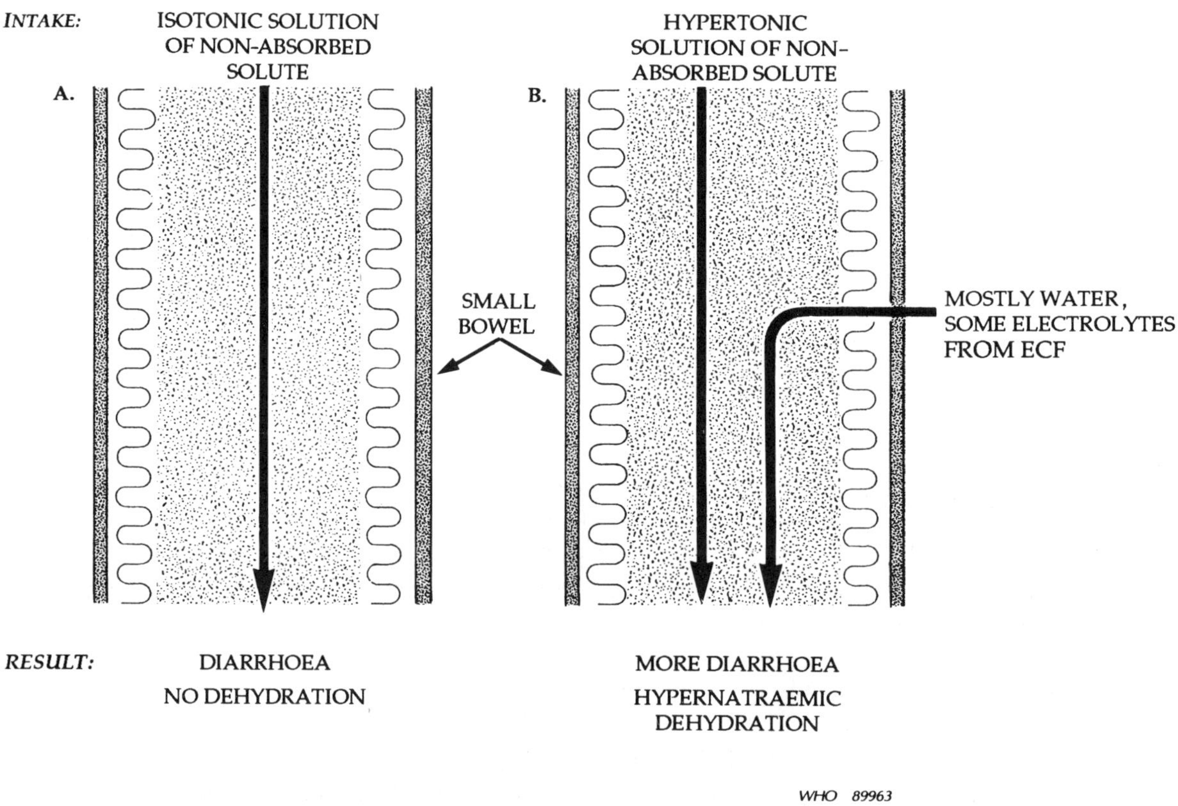

process may occur when the solute is lactose (in children with lactase deficiency) or glucose (in children with glucose malabsorption); both conditions are occasional complications of enteric infections. If the poorly absorbed substance is taken as a *hypertonic* solution, water (and some electrolytes) will move from the ECF into the gut lumen, until the osmolality of the intestinal contents equals that of the ECF and blood. This increases the volume of the stool and, more importantly, causes dehydration owing to the loss of body water (see Fig. 2.3, B). Because the loss of body water is greater than the loss of sodium chloride, hypernatraemia also develops (see below).

Consequences of watery diarrhoea

Patients with watery diarrhoea produce stools containing large amounts of sodium, chloride, potassium, and bicarbonate ions (see Table 2.1).

Table 2.1 **Electrolyte content of stool in acute watery diarrhoea and of oral rehydration salts solution**

	Average electrolyte content, mmol/l			
	Na^+	K^+	Cl^-	HCO_3^-
Cholera				
Adults	140	13	104	44
Children (below 5 years)	101	27	92	32
Non-cholera diarrhoea				
Children (below 5 years)	56	25	55	14
ORS solution	90	20	80	30[a]

[a] Or citrate, 10 mmol/l.

All the acute effects of watery diarrhoea are caused by the loss of water and electrolytes from the body in liquid stool. Additional amounts of water and electrolytes are lost when there is vomiting, and water losses are also increased by fever. These losses cause dehydration (due to the loss of water and sodium chloride), base-deficit acidosis (due to the loss of bicarbonate), and potassium depletion. Among these, dehydration is the most dangerous because it can cause decreased blood volume (hypovolaemia), cardiovascular collapse, and death if not treated promptly. Three types of dehydration are considered below.

Isotonic dehydration

This is the type of dehydration most frequently caused by diarrhoea. It occurs when the *net losses of water and sodium are in the same proportion* as normally found in the ECF. The principal features of isotonic dehydration are:

- there is a balanced deficit of water and sodium;
- serum sodium concentration is normal (130–150 mmol/l);
- serum osmolality is normal (275–295 mOsmol/l);
- hypovolaemia occurs as a result of a substantial loss of extracellular fluid.

Isotonic dehydration is manifested first by thirst, and subsequently by decreased skin turgor, tachycardia, dry mucous membranes, sunken eyes, lack of tears when crying, a sunken anterior fontanelle in infants, and oliguria. The physical signs of isotonic dehydration begin to appear when the fluid deficit approaches 5% of body weight and worsen as the deficit increases. As the fluid deficit approaches 10% of body weight, dehydration becomes severe, and anuria, hypotension, a feeble and very rapid radial pulse, cool and moist extremities, diminished consciousness, and other signs of hypovolaemic shock appear. A fluid deficit that exceeds 10% of body weight leads rapidly to death from circulatory collapse.

Hypertonic (hypernatraemic) dehydration

Some children with diarrhoea, especially young infants, develop hypernatraemic dehydration. This reflects a *net loss of water in excess of sodium*, when compared with the proportion normally found in ECF and blood. It usually results from the ingestion during diarrhoea of fluids that are hypertonic (owing to their content of sodium, sugar, or other osmotically active solutes) and not efficiently absorbed, and an insufficient intake of water or other low-solute drinks. The hypertonic fluids create an osmotic gradient that causes a flow of water from the ECF into the small intestine, leading to a decrease in the ECF volume and an increase in sodium concentration within the ECF (see Fig. 2.3, B). The principal features of hypernatraemic dehydration are:

- there is a deficit of water and sodium, but the deficit of water is greater;
- serum sodium concentration is elevated (>150 mmol/l);
- serum osmolality is elevated (>295 mOsmol/l);
- thirst is severe and out of proportion to the apparent degree of dehydration; the child is very irritable;
- seizures may occur, especially when the serum sodium concentration exceeds 165 mmol/l.

Hypotonic (hyponatraemic) dehydration

Children with diarrhoea who drink large amounts of water or other hypotonic fluids containing very low concentrations of salt and other solutes, or who receive intravenous infusions of 5% glucose in water, may develop hyponatraemia. This occurs because water is absorbed from the gut while the loss of salt (NaCl) continues, *causing a net loss of sodium in excess of water.* The principal features of hyponatraemic dehydration are:

- there is a deficit of water and sodium, but the deficit of sodium is greater;
- serum sodium concentration is low (<130 mmol/l);
- serum osmolality is low (<275 mOsmol/l);
- the child is lethargic; infrequently, there are seizures.

Base-deficit acidosis (metabolic acidosis)

During diarrhoea, a large amount of bicarbonate may be lost in the stool. If the kidneys continue to function normally, much of the lost bicarbonate is replaced and a serious base deficit does not develop. However, this compensating mechanism fails when renal function deteriorates, as happens when there is poor renal blood flow due to hypovolaemia. Then, base deficit and acidosis develop rapidly. Acidosis also results from excessive production of lactic acid when patients have hypovolaemic shock. The features of base-deficit acidosis include:

- serum bicarbonate concentration is reduced — it may be less than 10 mmol/l;
- arterial pH is reduced — it may be less than 7.10;
- breathing becomes deep and rapid, which helps to raise arterial pH by causing a compensating respiratory alkalosis;
- there is increased vomiting.

Hypokalaemia

Patients with diarrhoea often develop potassium depletion owing to large losses of potassium ion in the faeces; these losses are greatest in infants and can be especially dangerous in malnourished children, who are frequently potassium-deficient before diarrhoea starts. When potassium and bicarbonate are lost together, hypokalaemia does not usually develop. This is because the base-deficit acidosis that results from the loss of bicarbonate causes potassium to move from intracellular fluid to ECF in exchange for hydrogen ion, thus keeping the serum potassium level in a normal or even elevated range. However, when the base-deficit acidosis is corrected by giving bicarbonate, this shift is rapidly reversed, and serious hypokalaemia can develop. This can be prevented by replacing potassium and correcting the base deficit at the same time. The signs of hypokalaemia may include:

- general muscular weakness;
- cardiac arrhythmias;
- paralytic ileus, especially when drugs are taken that also depress peristalsis (such as opiates).

Rehydration therapy

The goal in managing dehydration caused by diarrhoea is to correct existing deficits of fluid and electrolytes rapidly (termed "rehydration therapy") and then to replace further losses as they occur until diarrhoea stops (termed "maintenance therapy"). Fluid losses can be replaced either orally or intravenously; the latter route is usually needed only for initial rehydration of patients who are severely dehydrated.

Oral rehydration therapy (ORT)

ORT is based on the principle that intestinal absorption of sodium (and thus of other electrolytes and water) is enhanced by the active absorption of certain food molecules such as glucose (which is derived from the breakdown of sucrose or cooked starches) or L-amino acids (which are derived from the breakdown of proteins and peptides) (see Fig. 2.2, D). Fortunately, this process continues to function normally during secretory diarrhoea, whereas other pathways of intestinal absorption of sodium are impaired. Thus, if patients with secretory diarrhoea drink an isotonic salt solution that does not contain a source of glucose or amino acids, sodium is not absorbed and the fluid remains in the gut, ultimately adding to the volume of stool passed by the patient (see

Fig. 2.4, A, B). However, when a balanced isotonic solution of glucose and salt is given, glucose-linked sodium absorption occurs and this is accompanied by the absorption of water and other electrolytes (see Fig. 2.2, D and Fig. 2.4, C). This process can correct existing deficits of water and electrolytes and replace further faecal losses in most

Fig. 2.4 **Effect of glucose on intestinal absorption of salt and water during diarrhoea**

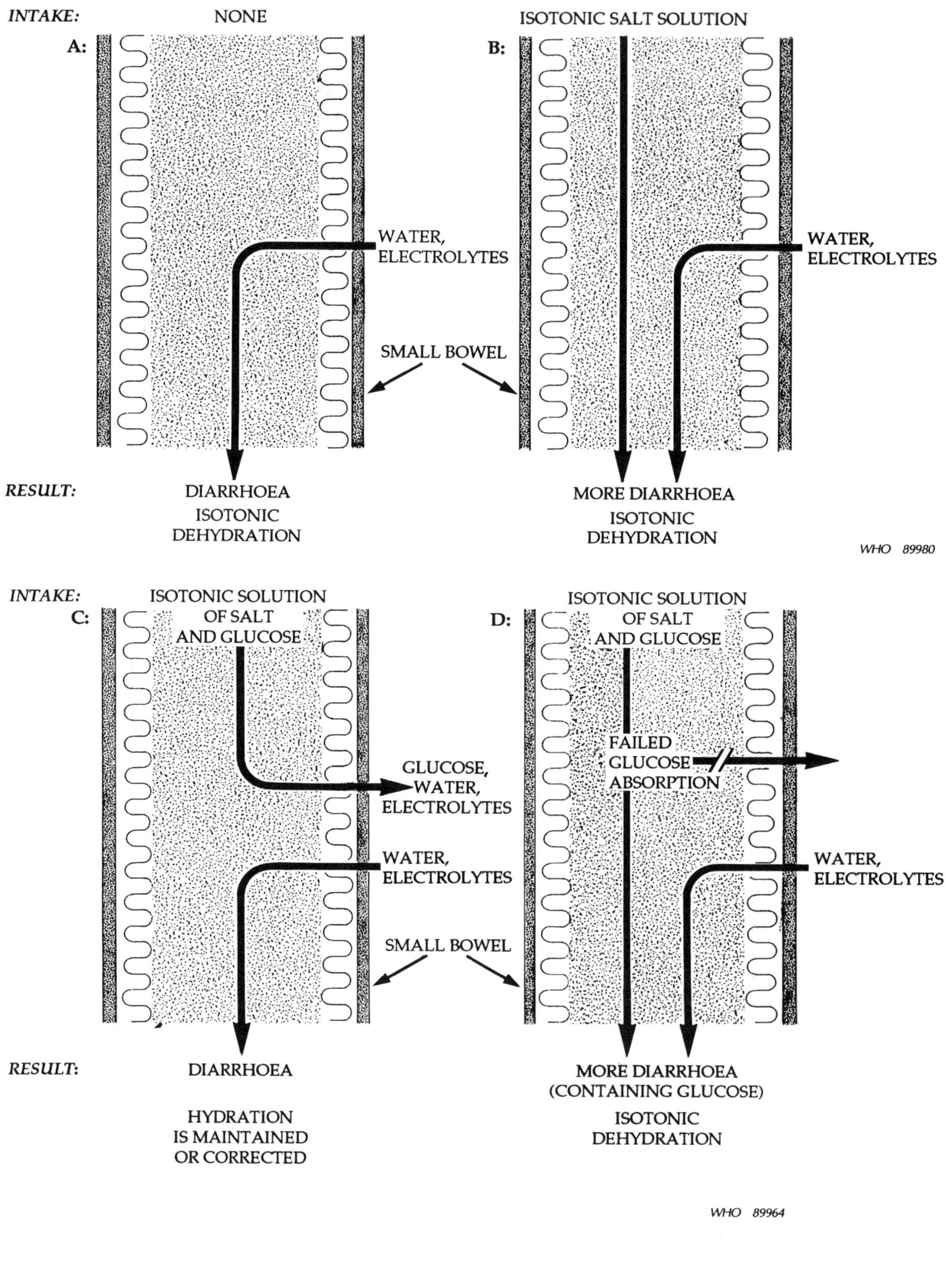

patients with secretory diarrhoea, irrespective of the cause of diarrhoea or the age of the patient.

Oral rehydration salts (ORS)

Composition of ORS. The principles underlying ORT have been applied to the development of a balanced mixture of glucose and electrolytes for use in treating and preventing dehydration, potassium depletion, and base deficit due to diarrhoea. To attain the latter two objectives, potassium and citrate (or bicarbonate) salts have been included, in addition to sodium chloride. This mixture of salts and glucose is termed *oral rehydration salts* (ORS); when ORS is dissolved in water, the mixture is called *ORS solution* (Table 2.2). The following guidelines were used in developing the WHO/UNICEF-recommended ORS solution:

- the solution should have an osmolality similar to, or less than, that of plasma, i.e. about 300 mOsmol/l or less;
- the concentration of sodium should be sufficient to replace efficiently the sodium deficit in children or adults with clinically significant dehydration;
- the ratio of glucose to sodium (in mmol/l) should be at least 1:1 to achieve maximum sodium absorption;
- the concentration of potassium should be about 20 mmol/l to replace potassium losses adequately;
- the concentration of base should be 10 mmol/l for citrate or 30 mmol/l for bicarbonate, which is satisfactory for correcting base-deficit acidosis due to diarrhoea. The use of trisodium citrate, dihydrate, is preferred, since this gives ORS packets a longer shelf-life.

Table 2.2 **Composition of the oral rehydration salts solution recommended by WHO and UNICEF**

Ingredients	**Amounts g/l**	**Ions**	**Concentration mmol/l**
Sodium chloride	3.5	Sodium	90
Trisodium citrate, dihydrate	2.9[a]	Potassium	20
Potassium chloride	1.5	Citrate	10[b]
		Chloride	80
Glucose (anhydrous)	20.0	Glucose	111

[a] Or 2.5 g sodium bicarbonate.
[b] Or 30 mmol bicarbonate.

Sodium concentration. ORS solution has been used to treat millions of cases of diarrhoea of different etiologies in patients of all ages, and has proved to be remarkably safe and effective. Nevertheless, because stool electrolyte concentrations vary in different types of diarrhoea and in patients of different ages, doctors are sometimes concerned about using a single ORS solution in all clinical situations. Table 2.1 (page 21) compares the composition of ORS solution with the average electrolyte composition of stool in different kinds of acute watery diarrhoea. The stools of patients with cholera contain relatively large amounts of sodium, potassium, and bicarbonate. In children with acute non-cholera diarrhoea, the concentrations of sodium, bicarbonate, and chloride in the stool are lower, although they vary considerably.

A child with dehydration due to diarrhoea has deficits of sodium and water. In cases of severe dehydration, the sodium deficit has been estimated to be 70–110 mmol for each 1000 ml deficit of water. The sodium concentration of 90 mmol/l in ORS solution is within this range and hence it is suitable for the treatment of dehydration. During the maintenance phase, however, when ORS solution is used to replace continuing losses of water and electrolytes in the stool, the concentration of sodium excreted in the stool averages 50 mmol/l. Although this loss could be corrected with a separate solution containing 50 mmol/l of sodium, the same result can be obtained by giving the standard ORS solution with a normal intake of water or breast milk. This approach reduces the average concentration of sodium ingested to a range that is both safe and effective, and any modest excess of sodium or water is excreted in the urine; this is especially important in young infants, in whom renal function is not fully developed. A major advantage of this approach is that it avoids confusing mothers, nurses, and doctors, who might otherwise have to use different oral solutions for the rehydration and maintenance phases of treatment.

Home fluids

Although their composition is not as appropriate as that of ORS solution for treating dehydration, other fluids such as soup, rice water, yoghurt drinks, or plain water may be more practical and nearly as effective for ORT to prevent dehydration. *These home fluids should be given to children to drink as soon as diarrhoea starts, with the goal of giving more fluid than usual.* Feeding should also be continued. Such early home therapy can prevent many patients from becoming dehydrated and it also facilitates continued feeding by restoring appetite.

Food-based fluids[1] are most effective for home therapy when they contain some salt; however, factors other than relative efficacy should be considered when recommending specific home fluids (see Unit 4). If fluids contain salt, the concentration of sodium should preferably be about 50 mmol/l. This concentration is obtained by dissolving 3.0 g of common salt in 1 litre of water. Fluids with higher salt concentrations may also be safe and effective, provided other salt-free fluids, such as water, are given.

Food-based fluids that contain starch are preferred to those containing sucrose, because they have a lower osmolality. Moreover, when starch is broken down within the intestine into glucose, it is rapidly absorbed. Thus, the osmolality of the fluid in the intestine remains at a safe level (i.e. less than 300 mOsm/l). A similar situation exists when a fluid contains proteins, e.g. soups made with legumes. The proteins break down slowly into amino acids, which are absorbed quickly, so that the osmolality of the fluid in the intestine remains within a safe range.

When only salt-free fluids are given, the diet should, if possible, contain some salted food. However, this combination is less effective in preventing dehydration when diarrhoea is severe; if given in large amounts without dietary salt, salt-free fluids might also cause hyponatraemia. Infants with diarrhoea should always continue to be breast-fed. Breast-feeding during diarrhoea is an important source of water and

[1] "Food-based" means that a fluid contains carbohydrates or proteins. It does not always mean that the fluid is made from food items such as yoghurt or cereals; fluids such as green coconut water are included as well.

nutrients, provides some salt, and can actually decrease stool volume and the duration of illness.

There are also some fluids that should not be given to children with diarrhoea. These include sweetened commercial fruit drinks or soft drinks, which are usually hyperosmolar owing to their high sucrose content. These fluids can cause osmotic diarrhoea and hypernatraemia. Other fluids to avoid are purgatives, and stimulants such as coffee.

Limitations of ORT

In at least 95% of episodes of watery diarrhoea, dehydration can be corrected or prevented using only ORS solution (or ORT). However, ORT is either inappropriate or ineffective in certain situations.

ORT is inappropriate for:

- initial treatment of severe (life-threatening) dehydration, because fluid must be replaced very rapidly (this requires intravenous infusion of water and electrolytes);
- patients with paralytic ileus and marked abdominal distension;
- patients who are unable to drink (however, ORS solution can be given to such patients through a nasogastric tube, if intravenous treatment is not possible).

ORT is ineffective for:

- patients with very rapid stool loss (> 15 ml/kg of body weight per hour); such patients may be unable to drink fluid at a sufficient rate to replace their losses;
- patients with severe, repeated vomiting (this is unusual); generally, most of the fluid taken orally is absorbed despite vomiting, and vomiting stops as dehydration and electrolyte imbalance are corrected;
- patients with glucose malabsorption (also unusual); in such cases ORS solution causes stool volume to increase markedly and the stool contains large amounts of glucose; dehydration may also worsen (see Fig. 2.4, D).

Intravenous therapy

Intravenous fluids are required only for patients with severe dehydration, and then only to restore rapidly their blood volume and correct hypovolaemic shock. Although a number of intravenous solutions are available, they are all deficient in at least some of the electrolytes required to correct the deficits found in patients dehydrated by acute diarrhoea (see Table 2.3). To ensure adequate electrolyte replacement, some ORS solution should be given as soon as the patient is able to drink, even while the initial fluid requirement is being provided by intravenous therapy. The following is a brief discussion of the relative merits of the most widely available solutions.

Preferred solution

Ringer's lactate solution (also called Hartmann's solution for injection) is the best commercially available solution. It supplies an adequate concentration of sodium and sufficient lactate, which is metabolized to bicarbonate, for the correction of base-deficit acidosis. However, the concentration of potassium is low and the solution provides no glucose to prevent hypoglycaemia. Ringer's lactate solution can be used

Table 2.3 **Electrolyte content of intravenous infusion solutions**

	Solution	Electrolyte content, mmol/l			
		Na^+	K^+	Cl^-	Lactate
A.	**Preferred**				
	Ringer's lactate (Hartmann's solution)	130	4	109	28
B.	**Acceptable**				
	Normal saline (9 g NaCl/l)	154	0	154	0
	Half-strength Darrow's solution	61	18	52	27
	Half-normal saline (4.5 g NaCl/l)	77	0	77	0
C.	**Unacceptable**				
	Glucose (dextrose) solutions	0	0	0	0

in all age groups to correct dehydration due to acute diarrhoea of any cause. Early provision of ORS solution and early resumption of feeding will provide the required amounts of potassium and glucose.

Acceptable solutions

When Ringer's lactate solution is not available, normal saline, half-strength Darrow's solution, or half-normal saline solution may be used; however, these are less appropriate as regards content of sodium, potassium, or a base precursor (see Table 2.3).

- *Normal saline* (also called isotonic or physiological saline) is often available. It does not contain a base to correct acidosis, nor does it replace potassium losses. Sodium bicarbonate or sodium lactate (20–30 mmol/l) and potassium chloride (5–15 mmol/l) can be added to the solution, but this requires a supply of the appropriate sterile solutions.

- *Half-strength Darrow's solution* (also called lactated potassic saline) contains less sodium chloride than is needed to correct efficiently the sodium deficit in patients with severe dehydration. It is prepared by diluting full-strength Darrow's solution with an equal volume of glucose solution (50 g/l or 100 g/l).

- *Half-normal saline* with 50 g or 100 g of glucose per litre, like normal saline, does not correct acidosis, nor does it replace potassium losses. It also contains less sodium chloride than is needed for optimal correction of dehydration.

Unacceptable solution

Plain glucose (dextrose) solution should *not* be used because it provides only water and glucose. It does not contain electrolytes and thus does not replace the electrolyte losses or correct acidosis. It does not effectively correct hypovolaemia.

Exercises

1. Indicate whether the following features are *most* characteristic of secretory or osmotic diarrhoea. Place an S (for secretory) or an O (for osmotic) against each, as appropriate.

   A. Hypernatraemic dehydration. ________________
   B. Isotonic dehydration. ________________
   C. Non-absorbed solute. ________________
   D. Impaired sodium absorption. ________________
   E. Lactose intolerance is a cause. ________________

2. Which of the following can increase the efficacy of sodium absorption in the small intestine? (There may be more than one correct answer.)

   A. Cooked rice starch.
   B. Palm oil.
   C. Plain sugar.
   D. Some amino acids.
   E. Glucose.

3. Which one of the following effects of severe diarrhoea is *most* dangerous?

   A. Potassium depletion.
   B. Anorexia.
   C. Base-deficit acidosis.
   D. Fever.
   E. Hypovolaemia.

4. Which of the following are features of hypertonic dehydration? (There may be more than one correct answer.)

   A. Extreme thirst.
   B. Serum sodium concentration: 140 mmol/l.
   C. Very irritable child.
   D. Serum potassium concentration: 3.8 mmol/l.
   E. Lethargic child.

5. For which of the following situations is ORT using ORS solution effective? (There may be more than one correct answer.)

   A. Maintenance therapy for an infant with diarrhoea due to rotavirus.
   B. Rehydration of a child with cholera who is alert and able to drink.
   C. Rehydration of a child with diarrhoea, paralytic ileus and abdominal distension.
   D. Rehydration of a comatose child with severe dehydration and shock due to rotavirus diarrhoea.
   E. Maintenance therapy of a child with cholera, after being rehydrated.

6. Which of the following might happen if ORS was mixed with only half of the required amount of water and used to treat a young child with rotavirus diarrhoea and

dehydration? (There may be more than one correct answer.)

A. The solution would be even more effective, causing the stool volume to be reduced and the duration of diarrhoea to be shortened.
B. The child would develop hypernatraemia.
C. The child would refuse to drink the solution.
D. The child would develop paralytic ileus and abdominal distension.
E. The child would become extremely thirsty.

7. Which of the following "home fluids" can be safely used to *prevent* dehydration in children with diarrhoea? (There may be more than one correct answer.)

A. Rice water.
B. Water.
C. Cola drink.
D. Soup made from cooked legumes.
E. Sweetened commercial fruit drink.

UNIT 3

Assessing the patient with diarrhoea

Introduction

Every child brought to a health facility because of diarrhoea should be carefully assessed before his or her treatment is planned. In most cases the information gained by spending a few minutes asking for details of the illness, and observing and examining the child for specific signs (e.g. of dehydration or malnutrition), is sufficient to make a diagnosis and develop a plan for treatment.

The clinical assessment consists of taking a brief history and examining the child. Its objectives are:

- to detect dehydration, if present, and determine its degree of severity;
- to diagnose dysentery, if present;
- to diagnose persistent diarrhoea, if present;
- to evaluate feeding practices and determine the child's nutritional status, especially to detect severe malnutrition;
- to diagnose any concurrent illness;
- to determine the child's immunization history, especially as regards immunization for measles.

Depending upon what is found, the clinical assessment should lead directly to:

- a plan for treating or preventing dehydration;
- a plan for treating dysentery, if present;
- a plan for treating persistent diarrhoea, if present;
- recommendations for feeding during and after diarrhoea;
- a plan for managing any concurrent illness;
- recommendations regarding measles immunization;
- a plan for follow-up.

This unit explains how the clinical assessment should be performed and interpreted, in order to ensure that the above objectives are achieved. Treatment plans for dehydration and other problems associated with diarrhoea, and for the maintenance of nutrition in patients with diarrhoea, are considered in Units 4–7.

Using the diarrhoea management chart and patient record form

The WHO chart "Management of the Patient with Diarrhoea" is designed to help guide the evaluation and treatment of patients with diarrhoea. It summarizes the questions to be asked and the signs to be observed in a manner that helps the doctor or health worker to remember the most important points and to follow a standard pattern in patient evaluation. It also shows how to use the results of the evaluation to determine the most appropriate treatment. This approach should be used for all children who are seen at a treatment facility with a complaint of *loose or watery stools* or *loose stools with blood.*

The top part of the chart shows how to assess patients for dehydration (Fig. 3.1), and how to assess and manage other important problems that patients with diarrhoea may have (Fig. 6.1, page 82). The clinical features described in these figures are the ones that are most important and can be most reliably assessed by doctors and other health workers.

Fig. 3.1 **How to assess patients for dehydration**

FIRST, ASSESS YOUR PATIENT FOR DEHYDRATION

		A	B	C
1. LOOK AT:	CONDITION	Well, alert	* **Restless, irritable** *	* **Lethargic or unconscious; floppy** *
	EYES	Normal	Sunken	Very sunken and dry
	TEARS	Present	Absent	Absent
	MOUTH and TONGUE	Moist	Dry	Very dry
	THIRST	Drinks normally, not thirsty	* **Thirsty, drinks eagerly** *	* **Drinks poorly or not able to drink** *
2. FEEL:	SKIN PINCH	Goes back quickly	* **Goes back slowly** *	* **Goes back very slowly** *
3. DECIDE:		The patient has NO SIGNS OF DEHYDRATION	If the patient has two or more signs including at least one * **sign** *, there is SOME DEHYDRATION	If the patient has two or more signs, including at least one * **sign** *, there is SEVERE DEHYDRATION
4. TREAT:		Use Treatment Plan A	Weigh the patient, if possible, and use Treatment Plan B	Weigh the patient and use Treatment Plan C URGENTLY

Information on the history, examination, and treatment of each patient should be summarized on a "patient record form". An example of such a form is given in Annex 1. Modified versions of this form may be used, but they should include at least:

- a brief history of the diarrhoeal episode, including its duration and whether blood has been seen in the faeces;
- the child's pre-illness feeding pattern;
- the child's immunization history, especially as regards measles;
- important findings during examination of the child, especially signs of dehydration or malnutrition, and the child's weight;
- a summary of fluid intake and output, and the evolution of clinical findings in patients given rehydration therapy at the health facility;
- a description of food given at the health facility;
- a description of any medicines given at the health facility;
- recommendations for treatment, feeding, and follow-up after the child leaves the health facility.

When the form is completed promptly and accurately, it provides a valuable record of the child's progress during treatment at the health facility. It also helps to remind the health worker of all the steps that should be taken in the evaluation and management of the patient. Completed forms should be kept at the health facility and reviewed regularly to identify areas in which case management practices could be improved. Forms completed by students should be checked by a supervising physician; this can serve as an important means of evaluating the student's skills in patient evaluation and case management.

Assessing the child for dehydration

Patients should first be evaluated for dehydration and then for other problems commonly associated with diarrhoea. Usually, both steps are completed before treatment is given. However, when a child is severely dehydrated, taking a complete history and doing a thorough examination must be deferred so that treatment can be started without delay. *Seeing a stuporous child, confirming that the condition began with diarrhoea and vomiting, and quickly confirming that the skin turgor is very poor give sufficient information to indicate that the patient has severe dehydration and requires an intravenous drip at once.* When the drip is running well, the history and physical examination should be completed.

Ask, look, and feel for signs of dehydration

The detection of dehydration is based entirely on *signs* observed when the child is examined. The signs that should be evaluated in every patient are as follows:

- *Condition and behaviour.* Carefully observe the child's general condition and behaviour. Does the child appear to be:

  —well, alert?
  —restless, irritable?
  —"floppy" (listless), lethargic, or unconscious?

Note that it is sometimes difficult to determine whether a child is abnormally lethargic or just sleepy. This can often be decided by asking the mother whether her child is lethargic or only sleepy.

- *Eyes*. Are the child's eyes:

  —normal?
  —sunken?
  —very sunken and dry?

Note that some children have eyes that are normally slightly sunken. It is often helpful to ask the mother whether her child's eyes are normal or more sunken than usual.

- *Tears*. Does the child have tears when he or she cries vigorously?

- *Mouth and tongue*. Are these:

  —wet?
  —dry?
  —very dry?

Note that this sign can be affected by events other than dehydration. The mouth and tongue will be moist if the child has been drinking or has recently vomited; they will be dry if the child is breathing through the mouth.

- *Thirst*. Offer the child some water or ORS solution in a cup or from a spoon and observe whether the child:

  —drinks normally, accepts the fluid without particular interest, or refuses to drink;
  —drinks eagerly, grasps the cup or spoon, or is unhappy when the fluid is removed;
  —is unable to drink or drinks poorly, because he or she is very lethargic or semiconscious.

- *Skin pinch (skin turgor)*. When the skin of the abdomen or thigh is pinched and released, does the fold flatten and disappear:

  —immediately?
  —slowly?
  —very slowly (i.e. taking more than 2 seconds)?

This sign is usually very helpful, but obese children may fail to show diminished skin turgor even when dehydrated, owing to the layer of fat under their skin, and skin turgor may appear poor in children with marasmus even when there is no dehydration (see Unit 7).

Additional signs that are not listed in Fig. 3.1 but can also be of help in assessing hydration include:

- *Anterior fontanelle*. In infants with some dehydration the anterior fontanelle is more sunken than usual; when dehydration is severe, it is very sunken.

- *Arms and legs*. The skin of the lower parts of the arms and legs is normally warm and dry; the colour of the nail beds is normally pink. When dehydration is severe and there is hypovolaemic shock, the skin becomes cool and moist, and the nail beds may be cyanosed.

- *Pulse*. As dehydration increases, the radial pulse and femoral pulse become more rapid. When dehydration is severe, the radial pulse becomes very rapid and weak. When there is hypovolaemic shock, it may disappear completely. The femoral pulse, however, remains palpable.

- *Breathing*. The rate of breathing is increased in children with severe dehydration, due in part to their base-deficit acidosis. The absence of cough or subcostal indrawing helps to differentiate these children from children with pneumonia.

The assessment of hydration status is difficult in children with *severe malnutrition* because many of the signs described above are altered by malnutrition. This is especially true for signs related to the child's general condition or behaviour, sunken eyes, absence of tears and diminished skin turgor. This topic is considered in greater detail in Unit 7.

Determine the degree of dehydration and select a Treatment Plan

After a patient with diarrhoea has been examined, the findings should be reviewed to determine the degree of dehydration (if any) and the appropriate Treatment Plan should be selected.

The signs that indicate dehydration are shown in Fig. 3.1, where they are organized into three columns (A, B, and C) according to the degree of severity. During the examination of the patient, each sign listed on the left of the figure should be evaluated and a circle placed around the descriptive term in column A, B, or C that best describes that sign in the patient. Signs that are most valuable in assessing dehydration, termed *"key signs"*, are marked with asterisks (*) and printed in **bold type**. Two or more circled signs in one column, *including at least one key sign*, mean that the patient falls in that category of dehydration and requires the corresponding Treatment Plan. If signs are noted in more than one column, as often occurs, the category of dehydration is the one farthest to the right (among columns A, B, and C) in which two items, *including at least one key sign*, are circled.

Column C—Severe dehydration

Look first at column C. If two or more signs are circled in that column, including at least one key sign, the patient has *severe dehydration*.

Patients with severe dehydration have a fluid deficit equal to more than 10% of their body weight. They are usually lethargic, stuporous or even comatose. The eyes are deeply sunken and without tears; the mouth and tongue are very dry, and breathing is rapid and deep. Patients who are awake are very thirsty; however, when there is stupor, the patient may drink poorly or be unable to drink. A skin pinch flattens very slowly (more than 2 seconds). The femoral pulse is very rapid and the radial pulse is either very rapid and feeble or undetectable. In infants the anterior fontanelle is very sunken. The patient may have passed no urine for 6 hours or longer. When there is hypovolaemic shock, the systolic blood pressure taken in the arm is low or undetectable, the arms and legs are cool and moist, and the nail beds may be cyanosed.

Severe dehydration requires urgent treatment with intravenous fluids, following Treatment Plan C (see Unit 5).

Column B — Some dehydration

If severe dehydration is not present, look next at column B. If two or more signs listed in that column are circled, including at least one key sign, the patient has *some dehydration*. Note that patients may have signs in both columns B and C. If the signs in column C are not sufficient to diagnose severe dehydration, they should be counted as belonging to column B.

Patients with some dehydration have a fluid deficit equal to 5–10% of their body weight. *This category includes both "mild" and "moderate" dehydration*, which are descriptive terms used in many textbooks:

- *"Mild" dehydration* (5–6% loss of body weight) is manifested mostly by increased thirst and restlessness. Skin turgor may be slightly decreased. Other signs associated with dehydration are not usually present.

- *"Moderate" dehydration* (7–10% loss of body weight) causes children to be restless, "fussy", or irritable. The eyes are somewhat sunken and the mouth and tongue are dry. There is increased thirst: older patients ask for water and young children drink eagerly when offered fluid from a cup or spoon. A skin pinch flattens somewhat slowly. The radial pulse is detectable, but rapid, and the anterior fontanelle in infants is more sunken than usual.

Patients with some dehydration should be treated with ORS solution given by mouth, following Treatment Plan B (see Unit 5).

Column A — No signs of dehydration

If neither severe dehydration nor some dehydration is present, conclude that the patient has *no signs of dehydration*.

Patients with diarrhoea but no signs of dehydration usually have a fluid deficit, but it equals less than 5% of their body weight. Although they lack distinct signs of dehydration, they should be given more fluid than usual to prevent signs of dehydration from developing.

Patients with no signs of dehydration should be treated at home, following Treatment Plan A (see Unit 4).

Weigh the child

Patients who are found to have *some dehydration* or *severe dehydration* should be weighed, if an accurate scale is available; children should be weighed unclothed. The body weight is important for determining the amount of oral or intravenous fluid to be given in Treatment Plans B and C (see Unit 5). If no scale is available, the body weight should be estimated on the basis of the child's age (see Fig. 5.1, page 66), and treatment should be given without delay.

The weight taken when a child is dehydrated should not be recorded on a growth chart, as it will be lower than normal owing to dehydration. Instead, the child should be reweighed after rehydration has been completed and that weight should be recorded on the chart. If possible, children with no signs of dehydration should also be weighed and the results recorded on their growth charts.

Assessing the child for other problems

After the patient has been evaluated for dehydration, other problems associated with diarrhoea should be considered. The assessment for other problems is summarized in Fig. 6.1 (page 82) and discussed below.

Dysentery

The health worker should ask whether the diarrhoea stools have contained any blood. If possible, a fresh stool specimen should also be examined for signs of blood. If blood is present, the patient should be considered to have *dysentery* and treated as described in Unit 6. If dehydration is present with the dysentery, it should also be treated immediately.

Persistent diarrhoea

The health worker should ask when the present episode of diarrhoea began. Episodes that have lasted at least 14 days should be considered to be *persistent diarrhoea* and treatment should follow the guidelines in Unit 6. Sometimes it is difficult to determine whether a child has persistent diarrhoea or is having sequential episodes of acute diarrhoea. Patients with persistent diarrhoea usually have loose stools every day, although the number per day may vary considerably. Sometimes, however, the child may have normal stools for 1 or 2 days after which diarrhoea resumes. *If the period of normal (formed) stools does not exceed 2 days, the illness should be considered a single diarrhoeal episode.* However, if the period of normal stools is longer than 2 days, any subsequent diarrhoea should be considered to be a new episode.

Malnutrition

A brief nutritional assessment should be carried out for each child with diarrhoea to identify those with nutritional problems and obtain the information necessary to make dietary recommendations. The minimum goals should be: (i) to determine whether the usual feeding pattern is appropriate for the child's age, and (ii) to detect severe malnutrition, if present. If conditions permit, a more thorough assessment should be performed as described below.

Feeding history

Determine both the child's usual (pre-illness) diet and the feeding pattern during the current episode of diarrhoea. The main points that follow should be covered. Examples of useful questions are provided for each point.

- *Pre-illness feeding:*

  —Breast-feeding
  Is the child breast-feeding?
  How frequently is breast milk given?
  If the child is less than 4–6 months of age, are any other liquids or food given?

  —Animal milk or infant formula
  Are either of these given?

  —For powdered milk or formula
  How is the milk prepared (i.e. how much powder and water)?
  Is boiled water used?
  How much milk is given and how often?
  Is the milk given in a feeding bottle, or by cup and spoon?

  —Solid foods (for children aged 4–6 months or older)
  What foods does the child usually take?
  Are the usual foods liquid, soft, or semi-solid?
  Is oil added to the child's food?
  How much food is given and how frequently?
  Is the child given food from the family pot?

- *Feeding during diarrhoea:*

  —Breast-feeding
  Is breast milk given more often, as usual, or less often?
  Does the child breast-feed well?

  —Animal milk or infant formula
  Has the amount given been more, the same, or less than usual?
  Has the milk or formula been made with more water than usual?

  —Other liquids
  Has the child been given water or other drinks?
  Has the amount of liquid given been more, the same, or less than usual?

  —Solid foods
  Has the amount given been more, the same, or less than usual?
  How frequently has food been offered?
  What types of food has the child accepted?

- *Mother's beliefs about feeding during diarrhoea:*

  —What does the mother believe about giving breast milk, animal milk or formula, other fluids or foods during diarrhoea?

—Which fluids or foods does she consider acceptable and which unacceptable during diarrhoea?

Physical findings

First, determine whether there is obvious severe protein–calorie malnutrition. This may have the features of marasmus, kwashiorkor, or both (see Fig. 3.2).

- *Signs of marasmus include:*

  —"old man's face";
  —extreme thinness, "skin and bones" appearance;
  —very thin extremities, distended abdomen;
  —absence of subcutaneous fat; the skin is very thin;
  —fretful, irritable behaviour.

- *Signs of kwashiorkor include:*

  —essential features:
  oedema;
  miserable, apathetic, listless behaviour;

  —other possible features:
  thin hair with reddish discoloration;
  flaking, dry skin;
  enlarged liver.

Then, determine whether there is a less serious degree of malnutrition. This may not be possible in all settings, but should be done where conditions permit. The following examinations may be performed:

- *Weight-for-age.* This is the simplest measure of nutritional status; however, it does not distinguish between past nutritional damage (i.e. stunting, which does not respond to increased feeding) and recent weight loss (i.e. wasting, for which increased feeding is important). Weight-for-age is most valuable when recorded on a growth chart and used to monitor *growth over time*; a series of points over several months shows whether or not the *growth pattern* is satisfactory (see Annex 2). Mothers of young children whose weight-for-age is below 70% of the standard, or whose weight is not increasing or is decreasing over time, should receive special nutritional advice. The children should be seen regularly for follow-up until a normal rate of growth is established.

- *Mid-upper arm circumference.* This test involves measurement of the circumference of the upper arm using a standard tape (see Annex 3). It is simple to perform (a weighing scale is not required) and valuable as a screening test for malnutrition. However, it is *not* useful for monitoring growth over time.

- *Weight-for-height/length.* A low weight-for-height ratio is valuable because it detects children with recent weight loss (wasting); however, two accurate measurements are required (i.e., weight and height/length). Unfortunately, height or length is more difficult to measure accurately than weight. Mothers of children whose

Fig. 3.2 **Clinical features of marasmus and kwashiorkor**

Marasmus

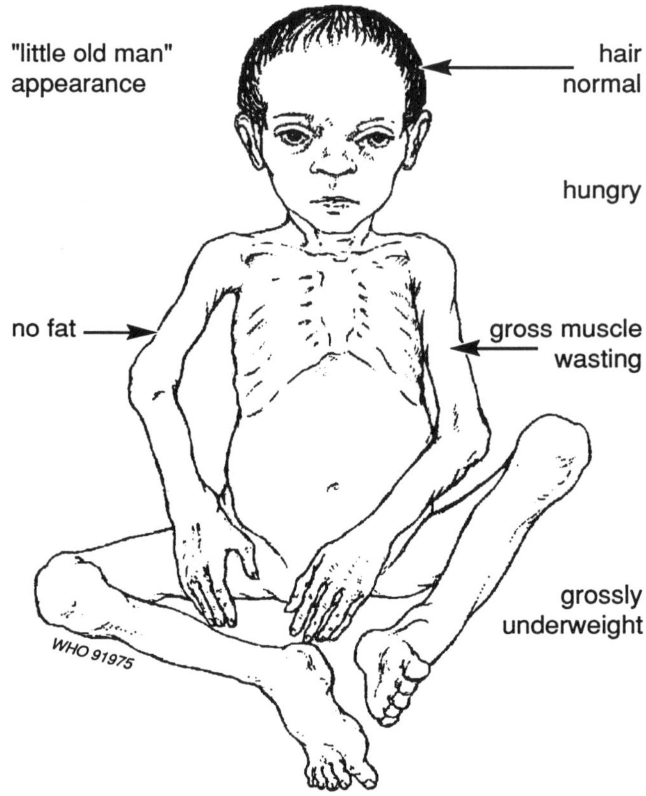

Kwashiorkor

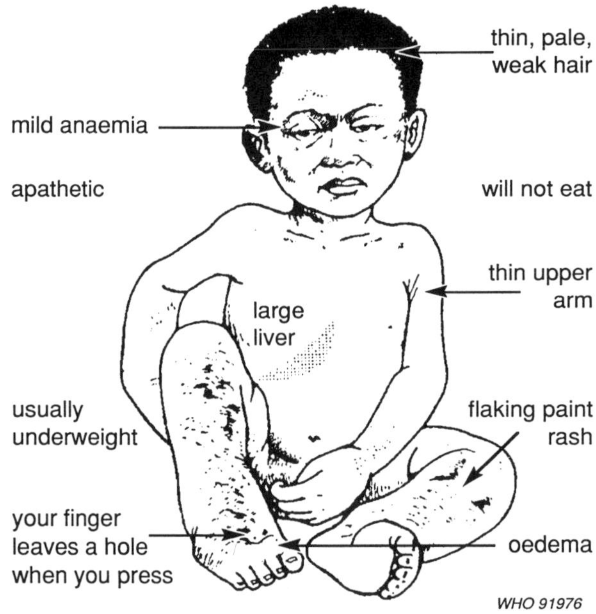

Source: King M. et al. *Primary child care. A manual for health workers. Book one.* Oxford, Oxford University Press, 1978.

weight-for-height ratio is below 75% of the standard should receive special nutritional advice and the children should be followed up.

Each of the above measurements should be interpreted using standard charts or tables. These may be either national or international standards. If the latter are used, national guidelines must be followed for their interpretation in the local setting.

Vitamin A deficiency

- *Night blindness.* Ask the mother if her child is able to see normally at night. Children with night blindness do not move about normally in the dark and may be unable to find their food or toys. Night blindness is difficult to recognize in children who are not yet old enough to walk.

- *Bitot's spots.* These are dry, grey-white, foamy-appearing areas, triangular in shape, located in the temporal part of the scleral conjunctiva. Usually both eyes are affected.

- *Corneal xerosis and ulceration.* These are areas of the cornea that are roughened or ulcerated.

Children who have night blindness, Bitot's spots, or corneal xerosis or ulceration should be treated immediately with therapeutic doses of vitamin A (see Unit 7).

Fever

The mother should be asked whether her child has had fever during the past 5 days. The child's temperature should also be measured. If rectal thermometers are available and can be disinfected after use, they are preferable. Otherwise, the temperature should be measured in the axilla (armpit). Any child with a history of recent fever or with a temperature of 38 °C or greater should be managed as described in Unit 6. Such children should also be carefully checked for signs or symptoms of other infections, e.g. pneumonia, malaria.

Measles vaccination status

The mother should be asked whether her child has been immunized against measles. The child's immunization record should also be consulted, if it is available. Children should receive measles vaccine at 9 months of age or as soon as possible thereafter. For unimmunized children, the best time to give the vaccine is during the child's current visit to the treatment facility.

Exercises

1. Which of the following are signs of *severe* dehydration?

   A. The skin pinch goes back slowly (within 2 seconds).
   B. The child is very lethargic.
   C. The child is unable to drink.
   D. The eyes are slightly sunken.
   E. The mouth and tongue are very dry.

2. Marina, aged 2 years, is brought to you because she has had diarrhoea for 3 days. When you examine her you note that she is irritable and fussy and that her skin

pinch goes back rather slowly. Other findings most consistent with her degree of dehydration would be:

A. Normal eyes, tears are present when she cries, and her mouth and tongue are moist.
B. Her eyes are very sunken, tears are absent when she cries, and she is unable to drink.
C. Her eyes are more sunken than usual, she drinks water eagerly from a cup, and her mouth and tongue are rather dry.
D. She has a fever (38.5 °C), her stool contains some blood, and she is not interested in drinking water.

3. A mother brings her 2-year-old daughter, Asita, to you because she has had diarrhoea for 2 days. When you examine her you note that she is irritable and fussy, her eyes are not sunken, she has tears when she cries, her mouth is somewhat dry, and she takes water eagerly from a cup. Her skin pinch goes back rather slowly. Asita does not appear to be malnourished.

Based on these findings, what conclusions would you draw about Asita's condition and how she should be treated? (There may be more than one correct answer.)

A. Asita has *severe dehydration.*
B. Asita has *no signs of dehydration.*
C. Asita has *some dehydration.*
D. Asita should be treated according to Treatment Plan A.
E. More information is needed to determine how Asita should be treated.

4. Bantu, aged 14 months, is brought to the health centre because of diarrhoea, which began 3 days ago. At first the stools were only loose, but yesterday his mother saw blood in them. She believes Bantu has a fever. He has also vomited two or three times. When you examine Bantu you note that he is alert, but irritable and restless. His eyes are not sunken, he has tears when he cries, his mouth is moist (but he has vomited recently), and he will drink some water, but not with much interest. His skin pinch goes back quickly. His temperature is 39 °C.

Which of the following statements are correct? (There may be more than one correct answer.)

A. Bantu has *some dehydration.*
B. Bantu should be treated for dysentery.
C. Bantu should be treated according to Treatment Plan B.
D. Bantu should be examined for possible infection outside the intestinal tract, e.g. pneumonia.
E. Bantu has *no signs of dehydration.*

5. Which of the following should be done *after* an 11-month-old child with diarrhoea has been assessed for possible dehydration? (There may be more than one correct answer.)

A. Ask whether there has been any blood in the stool.

B. Ask how long the diarrhoea has lasted.
C. Examine the child for signs of severe malnutrition.
D. Take the child's temperature.
E. Determine whether the child has received measles vaccine (and other recommended immunizations).

UNIT 4

Treatment of diarrhoea at home

Introduction

Home treatment is an essential part of the correct management of acute diarrhoea. This is because diarrhoea begins at home and children seen at a health facility will usually continue to have diarrhoea after returning home. Children must receive proper treatment at home if dehydration and nutritional damage are to be prevented. Mothers who are able to carry out home treatment should begin it *before* seeking medical care. When early home therapy is given, dehydration and nutritional damage can often be prevented.

Each mother whose child is treated for acute diarrhoea at a health facility should be taught how to continue the treatment of her child at home, and how to give early home therapy for future episodes of diarrhoea. When properly trained, mothers should be able to:

- prepare and give appropriate fluids for ORT;
- feed a child with diarrhoea correctly;
- recognize when a child should be taken to a health worker.

The steps involved in home therapy, the information and skills that mothers need to carry it out, and the ways in which these can be effectively communicated to them, are the subjects of this unit.

Treating diarrhoea at home — Treatment Plan A

The management of acute watery diarrhoea at home (Treatment Plan A) is outlined in Fig. 4.1. This plan should be used to treat children:

- who have been seen at a health facility and found to have *no signs of dehydration*;
- who have been treated at a health facility with Treatment Plan B or C until dehydration is corrected;
- who have recently developed diarrhoea, but have not visited a health facility.

The three basic rules of home therapy are considered below. These are:

- give the child more fluids than usual, to prevent dehydration;
- give the child plenty of nutritious food, to prevent malnutrition;
- take the child to a health facility if the diarrhoea does not get better, or if signs of dehydration or another serious illness develop.

Give the child more fluids than usual

Children with diarrhoea need more fluid than usual to replace that being lost in diarrhoeal stools and vomit. If suitable fluids are given in adequate volumes soon after diarrhoea starts, dehydration can often be prevented.

What fluids to give

Various home fluids can be given as early treatment to prevent dehydration. Many countries have specific recommendations, such as rice water, soup, yoghurt drinks,

Fig. 4.1 **Treatment Plan A: to treat diarrhoea at home**

TREATMENT PLAN A
TO TREAT DIARRHOEA AT HOME

USE THIS PLAN TO TEACH THE MOTHER TO:

- Continue to treat at home her child's current episode of diarrhoea.
- Give early treatment for future episodes of diarrhoea.

EXPLAIN THE THREE RULES FOR TREATING DIARRHOEA AT HOME:

1. **GIVE THE CHILD MORE FLUIDS THAN USUAL TO PREVENT DEHYDRATION:**
   - Use recommended home fluids. These include: ORS solution, food-based fluids (such as soup, rice water, and yoghurt drinks) and plain water. Use ORS solution for children described in the box below. (Note: If the child is under 6 months old and is not yet taking solid food, give ORS solution or water rather than a food-based fluid).
   - Give as much of these fluids as the child will take. Use the amounts shown below for ORS as a guide.
   - Continue giving these fluids until the diarrhoea stops.

2. **GIVE THE CHILD PLENTY OF FOOD TO PREVENT MALNUTRITION:**
   - Continue to breast-feed frequently.
   - If the child is not breast-fed, give the usual milk.
   - If the child is 6 months or older, or already taking solid food:
     - Also give cereal or another starchy food mixed, if possible, with pulses, vegetables, and meat or fish. Add 1 or 2 teaspoonfuls of vegetable oil to each serving.
     - Give fresh fruit juice or mashed banana to provide potassium.
     - Give freshly prepared foods. Cook and mash or grind food well.
     - Encourage the child to eat; offer food at least 6 times a day.
     - Give the same foods after diarrhoea stops, and give an extra meal each day for two weeks.

3. **TAKE THE CHILD TO THE HEALTH WORKER IF THE CHILD DOES NOT GET BETTER IN 3 DAYS OR DEVELOPS ANY OF THE FOLLOWING:**
   - Many watery stools
   - Repeated vomiting
   - Marked thirst
   - Eating or drinking poorly
   - Fever
   - Blood in the stool

CHILDREN SHOULD BE GIVEN ORS SOLUTION AT HOME, IF:

- *They have been on Treatment Plan B or C.*
- *They cannot return to the health worker if the diarrhoea gets worse.*
- *It is national policy to give ORS to all children who see a health worker for diarrhoea.*

IF THE CHILD WILL BE GIVEN ORS SOLUTION AT HOME, SHOW THE MOTHER HOW MUCH ORS TO GIVE AFTER EACH LOOSE STOOL AND GIVE HER ENOUGH PACKETS FOR 2 DAYS:

Age	Amount of ORS to give after each loose stool	Amount of ORS to provide for use at home
Less than 24 months	50-100 ml	500 ml/day
2 up to 10 years	100-200 ml	1000 ml/day
10 years or more	As much as wanted	2000 ml/day

- Describe and show the amount to be given after each stool using a local measure.

SHOW THE MOTHER HOW TO MIX ORS.

SHOW HER HOW TO GIVE ORS:

- Give a teaspoonful every 1-2 minutes for a child under 2 years.
- Give frequent sips from a cup for an older child.
- If the child vomits, wait 10 minutes. Then give the solution more slowly (for example, a spoonful every 2-3 minutes).
- If diarrhoea continues after the ORS packets are used up, tell the mother to give other fluids as described in the first rule above or return for more ORS.

and plain water; some recommend ORS solution. Although breast milk is considered a food, it is also an important home fluid and should be given freely.

In contrast, patients who have been treated for dehydration at a health facility should be given ORS solution at home until the diarrhoea stops (see Unit 5). Some countries also advise the use of ORS solution for home treatment of all patients seen at a health facility, including those with no signs of dehydration.

In all situations home fluids must meet certain criteria. The main points to remember are that home fluids must be:

- *Safe when given in large volumes.* Very sweet tea, soft drinks, and sweetened commercial fruit drinks, should be avoided. These are often hyperosmolar owing to their high sugar content (above 300 mOsm/l). They can cause osmotic diarrhoea, worsening dehydration and hypernatraemia. Also to be avoided are fluids with purgative action, and stimulants, such as coffee.

- *Easy to prepare.* The recipes for food-based fluids should be familiar and their preparation should not require much work or time. The required ingredients and measuring utensils should be readily available and inexpensive.

- *Acceptable.* The fluids should be ones that the mother is willing to give *freely* to a child with diarrhoea and that the child will readily accept.

- *Effective.* Fluids that are safe are also effective. However, some are more effective than others, depending upon their composition. Most effective are fluids that contain carbohydrate and protein, and some salt. However, nearly the same benefit may be obtained when water and other salt-free fluids are given freely along with weaning foods that contain salt.

The composition of home fluids is considered in Unit 2. Fluids suitable for home therapy are described below, in order of increasing efficacy:

- *Water.* Although water provides no salt or source of glucose, it is universally available and the idea of giving large volumes to a child with diarrhoea is generally accepted by mothers. Moreover, water is rapidly absorbed from the intestine and, when given with a diet that contains cooked cereals, preferably with added salt, would be adequate treatment for the majority of children with diarrhoea who are not dehydrated. Water should always be one of the fluids recommended for home therapy.

- *Food-based fluids.* Examples of food-based fluids are home-made soups, rice water or water in which other cereals have been cooked, and yoghurt-based drinks. These should be prepared in the traditional way and not diluted. The efficacy of these fluids can be increased by adding some salt (up to 3 g/l), but this requires special training of mothers, unless the fluid is normally prepared with salt, e.g. a vegetable soup.

- *Sugar–salt solution (SSS).* The composition of sugar–salt solution is nearly ideal for preventing dehydration. However, its preparation requires three correct measurements — sugar, salt and water — and mothers frequently have difficulty in remembering the recipe or in preparing the solution correctly; this may result in solutions that are hyperosmolar and unsafe. Other problems with sugar–salt solution are that sugar or salt may be unavailable, and mothers often give relatively small amounts of the fluid. For these reasons, many countries now recommend food-based fluids and water, as these do not require sucrose, do not involve a special recipe, and are less likely to be unsafe.

- *ORS solution.* Although not usually considered a "home fluid", ORS solution can be used in the home to prevent dehydration. Packets of ORS may be dispensed at health facilities for use at home, both to treat patients who have not become dehydrated and to continue the treatment of patients who have been rehydrated at the facility. Packets of ORS may also be available commercially for use in early home therapy. However, some commercial glucose–electrolyte products have compositions which differ appreciably from ORS and may be less satisfactory.

The selection of home fluids should usually be based on national recommendations. Factors to be considered when establishing recommendations include:

- *Importance of giving sufficient volume.* A major goal of home therapy is to give *more fluid than usual*, as much as the child will take. This is most likely to happen if *several fluids* are recommended, usually water and two or three familiar and acceptable food-based fluids.

- *Feasibility.* This includes such considerations as:

  —the availability to mothers of ingredients for food-based fluids;
  —the cost in time, effort and resources to teach mothers to prepare special recipes accurately and use the fluids correctly;
  —the availability of ORS and of an efficient system for its distribution, if ORS is selected for home use.

- *Age and feeding status.* Infants below 4–6 months of age who normally take only breast milk should not be given food-based fluids. They should be given only ORS solution or water, in addition to frequent breast-feeds.

- *Potential interference with proper feeding.* Home fluids that may interfere with efforts to teach good feeding practices during and after diarrhoea should not be used. For example, weaning foods (e.g. porridges) should not be diluted to prepare a home fluid, nor should dilute gruel or similar drinks be used when efforts are also being made to discourage their use as weaning foods because of their low nutrient content.

How much fluid and how often

Provide more fluid than usual. The general rule is to give the child as much fluid as he or she wants and to continue using ORT until diarrhoea stops. Remember that a child under 2 years of age cannot ask for something to drink; however, irritability and fussy behaviour are often signs of thirst. Young children must be *offered* fluids to determine whether they are thirsty and want to drink. When a child no longer accepts fluid, it is usually because enough has been taken to replace the losses caused by diarrhoea. Infants should be allowed to breast-feed as often and for as long as they want.

The following is a general guide for the amount of ORS solution or other fluid to be given at home after each loose stool:

- children under 2 years: 50–100 ml;
- children aged 2–10 years: 100–200 ml;
- children 10 years of age or older and adults should take as much as they want.

Show the mother how to measure the approximate amount of fluid to be given after each loose stool using a cup or some other container available to her at home (or that she can take home). Explain that the fluid should be given by teaspoon to children under 2 years of age: a teaspoonful every 1–2 minutes. Feeding bottles should *not* be used. Older children should take the fluid directly from a cup, by frequent sips. If vomiting occurs, the mother should stop giving the fluid for 10 minutes and then start again, but give it more slowly, e.g. one teaspoonful every 2–3 minutes.

If ORS solution is to be used at home, show the mother how to measure the correct amount of water, using a type of container available to her at home, and then how to mix the solution. Then give her enough packets to last 2 days. This should be enough to provide 500, 1000, or 2000 ml/day for children aged less than 2 years, 2–10 years, and 10 years or older and adults, respectively. When providing packets of ORS, explain to the mother that the *entire* packet must be mixed at one time and that any ORS solution that has not been used after 24 hours must be thrown away. Thus, if a packet makes 1 litre of solution, a child requiring 500 ml/day would still need two packets, one for each day. If diarrhoea continues after the packets have been used up, the mother should give the child the recommended home fluids or return to the health facility for more packets.

Give the child plenty of food

What foods to give

Breast-feeding should be continued without interruption. Formula or cow's milk should be given as usually prepared.

Children who are 6 months of age or older (and younger infants who have already begun to take soft foods) should also be given soft or semi-solid weaning foods. In general, such foods should provide at least half of the energy in the diet. If possible, salted foods should also be included, or weaning foods should be salted to taste. Guidelines concerning the type of foods to be given are shown in Fig. 4.1 and discussed in detail in Unit 7.

How much food and how often

During diarrhoea, give the child as much food as he or she wants. Offer food every 3–4 hours (six times a day). Small, frequent feedings are tolerated better than large feedings given less frequently. Many children have anorexia; they need to be coaxed to eat.

After the diarrhoea has stopped, give the child at least one more meal than usual each day for 2 weeks, using the same nutrient-rich foods that were given during diarrhoea; malnourished children should follow this regimen for a longer period (see Unit 7). The child should continue to receive these food mixtures as his or her regular diet, even after extra meals are no longer required.

"Antidiarrhoeal" drugs, antiemetics and antimicrobials

A wide variety of drugs and combinations of drugs are sold for the treatment of acute diarrhoea and vomiting. "Antidiarrhoeal" drugs include: antimotility agents (e.g. loperamide, diphenoxylate, codeine, tincture of opium), adsorbents (e.g. charcoal, kaolin, attapulgite, smectite), and live bacterial cultures (e.g. *Lactobacillus*, *Streptococcus faecalis*). Antiemetics include promethazine and chlorpromazine. *None* of these has been proved to have practical benefits for children with acute diarrhoea, and some may have dangerous side-effects. These drugs should *never* be given to children below 5 years of age.

Antimicrobials also should not be used routinely; they are of benefit *only* to patients with dysentery or suspected cholera and severe dehydration, and in selected patients with persistent diarrhoea (see Units 5 and 6). Antiprotozoal drugs are *rarely* indicated; their use is also described in Unit 6.

The overuse of antidiarrhoeal and antiemetic drugs, antimicrobials and antiprotozoal agents often delays the initiation of ORT or a visit to the health facility to seek help; it also wastes the precious financial resources of the family.

Problems in treating diarrhoea at home

The mother may encounter a variety of problems in treating her child with diarrhoea at home. Most of these can be avoided or solved by ensuring that she understands the importance of home treatment, is able to carry it out, knows what difficulties to expect, and receives constructive help and encouragement when problems arise. Table 4.1 describes some of the problems that are encountered most frequently and possible ways of solving or preventing them.

When to take the child to a health worker

The mother should be taught to watch for symptoms of worsening diarrhoea, dehydration, or other serious problems. Symptoms the mother can recognize include:

- the passage of many watery stools;
- repeated vomiting;
- increased thirst;
- failure to eat or drink normally.

Table 4.1 **Some difficulties encountered in home therapy for diarrhoea**

Difficulty	Possible solution
• The mother is disappointed because she is not given a prescription for drugs or the child does not receive an injection.	Explain that the diarrhoea will stop by itself after a few days. Also, explain that drugs do not help to stop diarrhoea, but that fluid replacement and continued feeding will help to shorten the illness and also maintain her child's strength and growth.
• The mother believes that food should not be given during diarrhoea.	Ask her to explain her beliefs about how diarrhoea should be treated. Discuss with her the importance of feeding in order to keep her child strong and support normal growth, even during diarrhoea.
• The mother does not know what fluids to give her child at home.	Ask her what fluids she can prepare at home and reach agreement on appropriate fluids for her child.
• The mother does not have the ingredients to make a recommended fluid.	Ask her if she can obtain the ingredients easily. If she cannot, suggest another home fluid.
• The child vomits after drinking ORS solution or other fluids.	Explain that more fluid is usually kept down than is vomited. Tell the mother to wait 10 minutes and then start giving fluid again, but more slowly.
• The child refuses to drink.	A child who has lost fluid will usually be thirsty and want to drink, even when there are no signs of dehydration. If the child is not familiar with the taste of ORS solution, some persuasion may be needed at first. When a child drinks well to begin with, then loses interest in drinking, it usually means that sufficient fluid has been given.
• The mother is given some packets of ORS for use at home but is afraid they will be used up before the diarrhoea stops.	Explain that after the ORS has been used up she should give a recommended home fluid (such as rice water) or water; or she could return to the health facility for more packets of ORS. In any event, she should continue to give extra fluid until the diarrhoea stops.

Children with dehydration may also be irritable and show no interest in playing. The mother should be instructed to bring her child to a health facility if the diarrhoea does not improve after 3 days, or if any of the symptoms described opposite appear. She should also bring the child if other problems develop, such as:

- fever;
- blood in the stool.

Talking with mothers about home treatment

Effective home treatment of diarrhoea can be given only by the child's mother (or other caregiver). It is she who must prepare the oral fluid and give it correctly, provide nutritious, well-prepared foods, and decide when the child needs to return to the treatment centre. The mother can do these tasks correctly only if she understands clearly what needs to be done and how to do it. The best opportunity for a mother to learn about home treatment of diarrhoea is when she brings her child to the treatment centre because the child has diarrhoea. Unfortunately, this opportunity is often lost because doctors or health workers do not communicate well with mothers; as a result, mothers frequently return home not understanding how to continue treating their children effectively.

There are a number of reasons why doctors often communicate poorly with mothers. For example, doctors have a "scientific" perspective and often speak in technical terms, they are authority figures, they are busy and have little time to spend with each mother, and they often "educate" mothers by *telling* them what to do. In contrast, the mother's perspective is usually traditional and unscientific, she does not understand technical terms, she may be easily frightened by authority figures, and she learns best through demonstration and practice in an atmosphere of patience, encouragement, and understanding.

A doctor who cannot communicate well with mothers will be ineffective in preparing them to carry out home treatment. To improve their communications with mothers, doctors (and other health workers) must learn:

- to listen to the mother and take her concerns seriously;
- to speak to her in terms she can understand;
- to be supportive and encouraging, giving her praise and help rather than criticism;
- to use teaching methods that require her active participation.

In real-life situations, doctors are rarely able to spend the time required to teach each mother how to carry out home treatment of diarrhoea: this must usually be done by other health workers. However, doctors must supervise this activity and this can only be done successfully if they themselves understand the principles of effective communication.

Some specific approaches that can be taken to improve communications with mothers and, especially, to help them to learn how to treat diarrhoea at home are considered below.

Using examples, demonstrations, and practice

Giving clear instructions on how to carry out home treatment is important, but represents only the first step in the training of mothers. Combining instruction with the use of examples, demonstrations, and practice can greatly facilitate the learning process. For instance, a health worker teaching a mother how to carry out ORT at home can make the message clearer by showing her a half-cup (100 ml) of ORS solution (with a line marking the appropriate level) while instructing her to give her child that amount after each loose stool. Or, a mother could be encouraged to watch another mother giving an infant ORS solution with a spoon so that she can see how to hold her child and how frequently to give the spoonfuls of fluid. She should then practise giving ORS solution to her own child, with guidance from the health worker. In this way, the health worker can see which parts of the task the mother finds difficult, and can explain or demonstrate how they should be done. Once the mother has performed the task correctly, the health worker can be confident that she has learned it.

Examples, demonstrations, and practice may include:

- *Showing pictures*: use a drawing or a poster of a mother breast-feeding while discussing the importance of this practice for an infant's health.

- *Using specific names or instructions* appropriate to local circumstances (instead of stating a general rule): advise the mother to give "banana or green coconut water" (which are rich in potassium), instead of simply telling her to give her child "fruit"; explain that she should feed her child "six times a day" instead of "frequently" or "more often than usual".

- *Demonstrating a task*: show the mother how to measure the correct amount of water for preparing ORS solution, using a container of a type that is available to her at home.

- *Showing an object*: show the mother an infant feeding bottle when explaining that this should not be used for giving milk or other fluids to her infant. Show a cup and spoon for comparison.

- *Telling a story*: a story of how another mother dealt with problems that arose while treating her child at home can help to prepare a mother for difficulties she may have to face. Stress that giving food and fluids will keep the baby strong and help the baby to continue growing, even while he or she has diarrhoea.

- *Practising a procedure*: let the mother practise preparing and giving ORS solution to her child using a cup and spoon.

Asking checking questions

Asking simple checking questions is a very effective way of confirming what a mother has learned about home therapy. For example, after explaining how to treat the child's diarrhoea at home, the doctor might ask: "Describe how you would prepare the drink for Ana" or "Tell me the symptoms that mean you should bring Ana back to me".

A checking question should be phrased in such a way that the answer cannot be just "yes" or "no". For example, it is not effective to ask: "Do you understand the symptoms that mean you should bring Ana back to see me?" The mother is likely to answer "yes", whether she understands them or not.

If a nurse or other staff member is responsible for teaching mothers, checking questions can be used to monitor his or her effectiveness. For example:

3-year-old Mo was treated for dehydration and is now ready to go home. The nurse has talked to his mother about what she should do at home to care for Mo.

The doctor should not ask the mother, "Did the nurse explain to you how to mix ORS solution?", or "Do you know how to mix ORS solution?", since the mother would probably be reluctant to answer "no". Instead, the doctor should ask questions such as "How much water will you mix with that ORS packet?", "How much of the solution will you give to Mo?", "How long did the nurse tell you to continue giving the ORS solution?", "What else will you give him to eat and drink?", and "When will you bring Mo back to see the nurse again?"

Providing illustrated instruction leaflets

A specifically prepared pamphlet (or card) can greatly improve communication with the mother. It should summarize the important elements of caring for a child with diarrhoea at home, and should have words and pictures that illustrate these points. When a pamphlet is being developed, it should be carefully tested to determine whether mothers understand its messages. An example of the possible content and layout of a mother's pamphlet is shown in Fig. 4.2.

There are many reasons why a mother's pamphlet is useful. For example:

- The pamphlet will simplify the task of training health workers in the messages to tell mothers.
- Referring to the pamphlet will bring to mind the main points to be covered when giving instructions to mothers.
- When she is at home, the pamphlet will remind the mother of what she was taught at the treatment facility, and support her if other family members or friends should disagree with her treatment.
- Mothers who cannot read will find the pictures helpful; otherwise a family member or neighbour can read out the written instructions, and learn from the pamphlet too.
- If the mother keeps the pamphlet, the next time her child has diarrhoea she can refer to it and remind herself what to do.
- The mother will appreciate being given something during her visit, especially if she is not given a medicine for the child.

Giving encouragement and assistance

Using examples, demonstrations, and a mother's pamphlet, and asking checking questions can help to ensure that a mother understands home therapy, but they do not guarantee that she will practise it. There are a number of reasons why a mother may not carry out the instructions received at a health facility. For example:

- Home treatment may seem to be unrewarding:
  - —she may expect ORT to stop the diarrhoea, and be discouraged when it does not;
  - —ORT may appear to have undesirable effects, such as making the child vomit more;
  - —home treatment is time-consuming and may be difficult: coaxing a sick child to eat can be frustrating.
- The necessary materials for ORT are not available: she may not have salt at home or a container to measure water.

Fig. 4.2 **How to treat diarrhoea at home (mother's pamphlet)**

AS SOON AS DIARRHOEA STARTS, GIVE YOUR CHILD MORE FLUIDS THAN USUAL:

IVE:

ORS solution

Food-based fluids, such as soup, rice water and yoghurt drink

Plain water

If the child is under 6 months old and taking only breast milk, give only ORS solution or plain water, in addition to breast milk.

IVE AS MUCH OF THESE FLUIDS AS YOUR HILD WANTS.

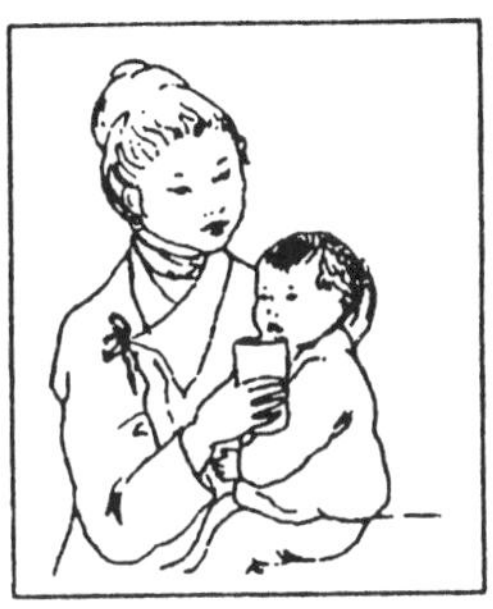

2. GIVE YOUR CHILD PLENTY OF FOOD

- Breast-feed frequently.
- If not breast-feeding, give the usual milk.
- If your child is 6 months or older, or already taking solid food, also give:
  - cereal or another starchy food mixed with pulses, vegetables, meat or fish, and a little oil
  - fresh fruit juice or mashed banana
  - freshly prepared foods, cooked and mashed or ground well
  - frequent, small meals (at least 6 per day)
  - an extra meal each day for 2 weeks after diarrhoea stops.

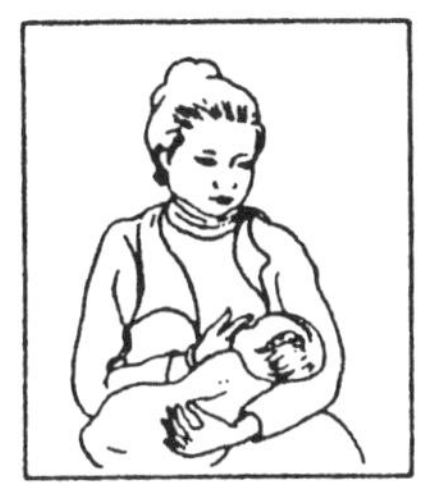

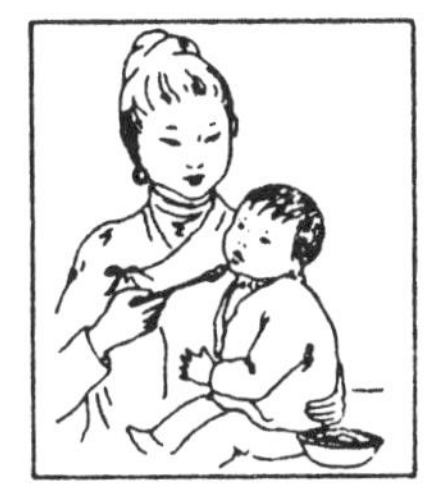

TAKE YOUR CHILD TO THE HEALTH WORKER IF THE CHILD:

Does not get better in 3 days

Passes many watery stools

Vomits repeatedly

Is very thirsty

Eats or drinks poorly

Has a fever

Has blood in the stool.

O NOT GIVE DRUGS FOR DIARRHOEA NLESS RECOMMENDED BY A HEALTH WORKER

4. YOU CAN PREVENT DIARRHOEA BY:

- Giving only breast milk for the first 4-6 months and continuing to breast-feed for at least 2 years
- Starting foods listed in section 2 of this card at 4-6 months
- Giving freshly prepared foods and clean drinking water
- Giving milk and other fluids by cup and spoon instead of feeding bottle
- Having all family members wash hands after passing stools and before preparing or eating food
- Having all family members use a latrine
- Putting a young child's stools in a latrine or burying them
- Having your child immunized against measles at the recommended age.

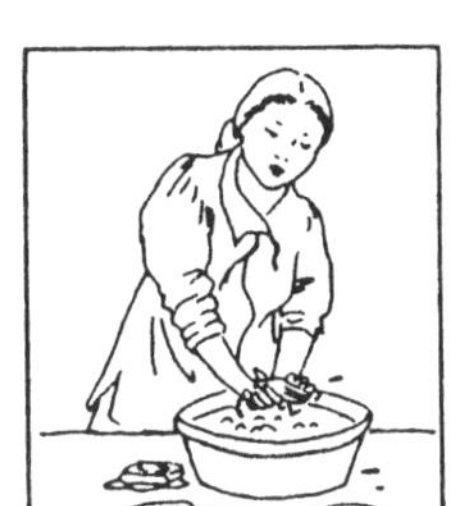

These problems can best be overcome by giving the mother encouragement and support. Several approaches should be used:

- *Emphasize the positive.* Explain that ORT will make the child stronger and that continued feeding will help the child to grow. Encourage the mother to look at the whole child, not just the child's stools. The child should be less fussy and more contented after ORT and feeding. Explain that, so long as this is the case, her treatment is successful and the diarrhoea will soon stop.

- *Give praise.* Praise is essential in building up a mother's confidence that she can treat her child successfully at home. Opportunities to praise the mother occur when she answers a checking question correctly, performs a practical task correctly (even if guidance was provided), or replies correctly on aspects of diarrhoea management at home, such as continued feeding.

- *Show interest.* Discuss with the mother how she will practise home therapy. Ask, for example, "What foods will you give your child?" When the mother answers, confirm that the food is suitable, or suggest another choice. Also discuss how she will prepare the food. By showing interest, the health worker will reinforce the mother's commitment to carry out treatment recommendations.

- *Assist with problems.* Ask questions to determine whether the mother has the necessary items for home therapy, e.g. a container to measure water. If the items are not available, suggest how they might be obtained.

- *Avoid giving too much information at one time.* Teach the mother only what she can remember and use. It is most important that mothers understand what fluids and food to give at home, and what signs mean they should bring the child back to the health centre. Messages on how to prevent diarrhoea should usually be reserved for mothers who already know how to treat their child at home.

Exercises

1. A mother has brought her 11-month-old daughter to a health centre because the child has diarrhoea. The mother breast-feeds the child. She says she lives far from the health centre and might not be able to come back for several days, even if the child gets worse. The mother mentions that she usually gives her child weak tea when she has diarrhoea, but has heard that the health centre has something better.

   The health worker assesses the child for signs of dehydration, but finds none. He decides to treat the child according to Treatment Plan A. Which of the following steps should the health worker take? (There may be more than one correct answer.)

   A. Advise the mother to continue breast-feeding the child as often and as long as the child wants.
   B. Give the mother enough packets of ORS to last 2 days. Show her how to prepare ORS solution and how much to give after each loose stool.
   C. Advise the mother to give her daughter rice with added vegetable oil, well-cooked vegetables, and, if possible, some well-ground meat, in addition to breast milk. These should be given in small feedings, at least six times a day.

D. Explain that, if the diarrhoea continues after the ORS has been used up, she should give rice water (or another recommended home fluid) in its place, while continuing to give breast milk and other foods.
E. Explain that if the diarrhoea continues for 3–4 days, she should discontinue breast-feeding until it stops.

2. Which of the following fluids are acceptable for ORT at home? (There may be more than one correct answer.)

A. Water.
B. Rice water.
C. A sweetened commercial fruit drink.
D. Soup.
E. A soft drink.

3. Harish, aged 9 months, has had watery diarrhoea for 2 days. He has been weaned and takes a mixed diet of rice, pulses, vegetables, and cow's milk. During the illness, however, his mother has given him only soft, boiled rice and tea. She has also obtained a medicine from the chemist which is given to stop the diarrhoea. When seen at the health centre, Harish has no signs of dehydration and is well nourished. Which of the following recommendations are appropriate? (There may be more than one correct answer.)

A. The mother should be encouraged to give Harish extra fluids at home, for example some soup or rice water after each watery stool.
B. The medication obtained from the chemist should be stopped.
C. Harish should resume his normal diet.
D. Harish should be brought back to the clinic if he does not eat or drink normally at home, or if he starts to pass many watery stools.

4. Juma, a 14-month-old boy, has had diarrhoea for 3 days and has been assessed as having some dehydration. He has been treated with ORS solution at the clinic, his signs of dehydration have disappeared, and he is now ready to go home. The doctor wishes to do everything possible to ensure that Juma will be well treated at home and will not need to return to the clinic. Which of the following steps would be appropriate? (There may be more than one correct answer.)

A. Give Juma's mother enough packets of ORS for 2 days, show her how to prepare and give ORS solution, and explain how much should be given after each loose stool.
B. Give Juma an antimicrobial to help stop his diarrhoea.
C. Explain to Juma's mother the importance of continuing to give him plenty of food.
D. Teach Juma's mother the symptoms that mean she should bring him back to the clinic.

5. If a mother is to be successful in carrying out ORT at home, it is important that she learns how this is done. Which one of the following methods is *most* effective in teaching mothers how to give ORT?

   A. The doctor explains how it is done.
   B. Posters on the clinic walls show how ORT is given.
   C. A nurse or health worker demonstrates ORT.
   D. The mother practises giving ORT with the guidance of a health worker.
   E. The mother is given an illustrated pamphlet that explains how ORT is carried out.

UNIT 5

Treatment of dehydrated patients

Introduction

Dehydration occurs when the water and electrolytes lost during diarrhoea are not fully replaced. As dehydration develops, various signs and symptoms appear which can be used to estimate the extent of dehydration and guide therapy. Three categories of dehydration can be recognized, each of which is associated with a specific treatment plan (see Unit 3). In increasing order of severity, these are:

- *No signs of dehydration* — follow Treatment Plan A
  Patients in this category have a fluid deficit equal to less than 5% of their body weight.
- *Some dehydration* — follow Treatment Plan B
  Patients in this category have a fluid deficit equal to 5–10% of their body weight.
- *Severe dehydration* — follow Treatment Plan C
  Patients in this category have a fluid deficit equal to more than 10% of their body weight.

Treatment Plan A (for treatment of diarrhoea at home) is described in Unit 4. This unit describes the treatment at a health facility of infants and children with *some dehydration* or *severe dehydration*, using Treatment Plans B and C, respectively.

Treatment of patients with some dehydration — Treatment Plan B

Children with signs indicating that there is *some dehydration* usually do not need to be admitted to hospital. They can be treated in a special area of the clinic known as the "ORT corner" or the "oral rehydration area". Mothers should stay with their children to help with the treatment and learn how to continue it at home, after the child is rehydrated.

Tasks involved in Treatment Plan B

The main tasks of Treatment Plan B (Fig. 5.1) are:

- to estimate the amount of ORS solution to be given during the first 4 hours, for rehydration;
- to show the mother how to give ORS solution;
- to continue breast-feeding and give other fluids, as required;
- to monitor treatment and reassess the child periodically until rehydration is completed;
- to identify patients who cannot be treated satisfactorily with ORS solution by mouth and adopt a more appropriate method of treatment;
- to give instructions for continuing the treatment at home after rehydration is completed, following Treatment Plan A.

How much ORS solution should be given?

When there is some dehydration the deficit of water is between 50 and 100 ml for each kg of body weight. If the child's weight is known, the amount of ORS solution required

Fig. 5.1 **Treatment Plan B: for patients with some dehydration**

TREATMENT PLAN B TO TREAT DEHYDRATION

APPROXIMATE AMOUNT OF ORS SOLUTION TO GIVE IN THE FIRST 4 HOURS:

Age: *	Less than 4 months	4 - 11 months	12 - 23 months	2 - 4 years	5 - 14 years	15 years or older
Weight:	Less than 5 kg	5 - 7.9 kg	8 - 10.9 kg	11 - 15.9 kg	16 - 29.9 kg	30 kg or more
in ml	200-400	400-600	600-800	800-1200	1200-2200	2200-4000
in local measure						

* Use the patient's age only when you do not know the weight. The approximate amount of ORS required (in ml) can also be calculated by multiplying the patient's weight (in kg) times 75.

- If the child wants more ORS than shown, give more.
- Encourage the mother to continue breast-feeding.
- For infants under 6 months who are not breast-fed, also give 100-200 ml clean water during this period.

OBSERVE THE CHILD CAREFULLY AND HELP THE MOTHER GIVE ORS SOLUTION:

- Show her how much solution to give her child.
- Show her how to give it - a teaspoonful every 1-2 minutes for a child under 2 years, frequent sips from a cup for an older child.
- Check from time to time to see if there are problems.
- If the child vomits, wait 10 minutes and then continue giving ORS, but more slowly, for example, a spoonful every 2-3 minutes.
- If the child's eyelids become puffy, stop ORS and give plain water or breast milk. Give ORS according to Plan A when the puffiness is gone.

AFTER 4 HOURS, REASSESS THE CHILD USING THE ASSESSMENT CHART. THEN SELECT PLAN A, B, OR C TO CONTINUE TREATMENT.

- If there are **no signs of dehydration**, shift to Plan A. When dehydration has been corrected, the child usually passes urine and may also be tired and fall asleep.
- If signs indicating **some dehydration** are still present, repeat Plan B, but start to offer food, milk and juice as described in Plan A.
- If signs indicating **severe dehydration** have appeared, shift to Plan C.

IF THE MOTHER MUST LEAVE BEFORE COMPLETING TREATMENT PLAN B:

- Show her how much ORS to give to finish the 4-hour treatment at home.
- Give her enough ORS packets to complete rehydration, and for 2 more days as shown in Plan A.
- Show her how to prepare ORS solution.
- Explain to her the three rules in Plan A for treating her child at home:
  - to give ORS or other fluids until diarrhoea stops
  - to feed the child
  - to bring the child back to the health worker, if necessary.

for rehydration can be estimated, using 75 ml/kg as the approximate deficit. The approximate volume of ORS solution (in ml) can be calculated by multiplying the weight (in kilograms) by 75. Thus, a child weighing 8 kg would require about 600 ml (i.e. 8 × 75) of ORS solution. If the child's weight is not known, the estimated deficit can be determined using the child's age, although this approach is less precise. Both methods are shown in Fig. 5.1, which indicates the range of fluid volumes that is usually appropriate for a child of a given weight or age.

It should be emphasized that the range of fluid volumes shown in the table is an *estimate* of what is needed and should be used only as a guide. The actual amount given should be determined by how thirsty the patient is and by monitoring the signs of dehydration, bearing in mind that larger volumes will be required by larger patients, those with more advanced signs of dehydration, and those who continue to pass watery stools during rehydration. The general rule is that patients should be given as much ORS solution as they will drink, and the signs of dehydration should be monitored to confirm that they are improving.

Giving ORS solution and other fluids

The estimated amount of ORS solution to be given during the first 4 hours should be explained to the mother, using measuring units with which she is familiar, e.g. 4 cups, 2 glasses, etc.

Fig. 5.2 **Using a cup and spoon to give ORS solution to a young child**

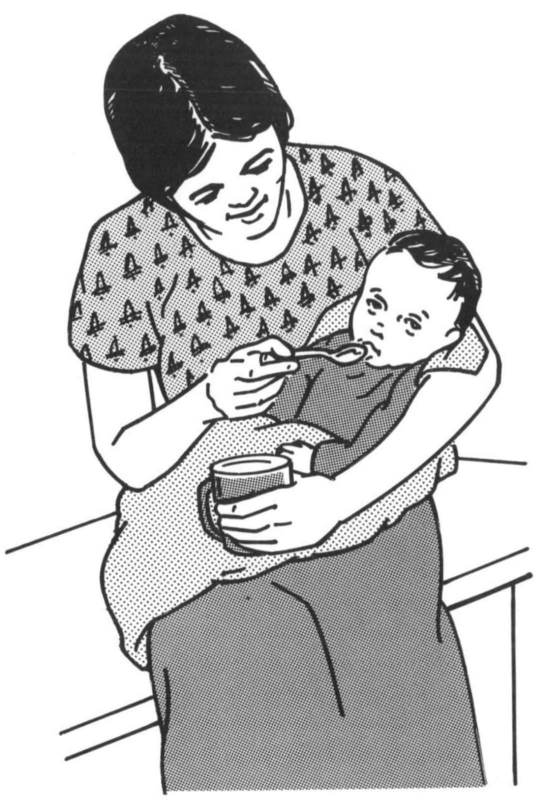

The mother should then learn how to give ORS solution to her child (Fig. 5.2). This is best done by means of a brief demonstration by a nurse or health worker, following which the mother should give her child the solution, under supervision, observing the following guidelines:

- Give one teaspoonful every 1–2 minutes to children under 2 years of age, or offer frequent sips from a cup to older children. Adults may drink the solution freely. Try to give the estimated amount of ORS solution in 4 hours.
- If the child vomits, wait 10 minutes, then continue giving ORS solution, but more slowly: one teaspoonful every 2–3 minutes.
- If the child will drink more than the estimated amount of ORS solution and is not vomiting, give more; if the child refuses to drink the estimated amount, *and the signs of dehydration have disappeared*, rehydration is completed: shift to Treatment Plan A.
- If the child normally breast-feeds, continue breast-feeding during therapy with ORS solution.
- For infants under 6 months of age who are not breast-fed, also give 100–200 ml of clean water during the first 4 hours.

When the mother has learned to give the fluid and the child is taking it well, she should be shown how to prepare ORS solution using containers of a type available in her home or that she can obtain easily. The health worker should demonstrate the method by mixing a packet. Then the mother should prepare the solution herself to ensure that she understands.

Monitoring treatment

During rehydration with ORS solution the child's treatment and progress should be monitored as follows:

- Check regularly to be certain that the mother is giving ORS solution correctly and the child is taking it satisfactorily.

- Record the amount of solution taken and the number of diarrhoea stools passed.

- Watch for problems, such as signs of worsening dehydration (e.g. further loss of skin turgor, increasing lethargy) or increasing stool output, which may indicate that ORT will not be successful. The management of such patients is discussed later in this unit.

- Watch for puffy eyelids, which are a sign of overhydration; if these are seen, treatment with ORS solution should be stopped, although breast-feeding and the provision of plain water should continue. When the puffiness is gone, the child should be considered to be rehydrated and further treatment should follow Treatment Plan A.

Reassessing the patient

After 4 hours, carefully reassess the child's hydration status following the assessment chart in Fig. 3.1 (page 34):

- If the child has *no signs of dehydration*, rehydration is complete. The child may be sent home after a health worker has carefully shown the mother how to continue treatment at home with ORS solution and feeding following Treatment Plan A, given her enough packets of ORS for 2 days, and explained the signs that mean the child should return to the health centre (see Unit 4).

- If signs indicating *some dehydration* are still present, continue rehydration therapy by again giving the volume of ORS solution estimated from Treatment Plan B. Continue this approach until the signs of dehydration have disappeared. Also start to offer food and drink as described in Treatment Plan A.

- If the child is passing watery stools frequently and the *signs of dehydration have worsened*, ORT should be temporarily stopped and the child rehydrated intravenously as described in Treatment Plan C (see Fig. 5.3).

Patients who cannot remain at the treatment centre

If the mother must leave *before* rehydration therapy is completed:

- Show her how much ORS solution to give the child to complete the initial 4-hour treatment at home. If possible, she should make up some solution under supervision and give it during the journey.

- Give her enough packets of ORS to complete the initial rehydration *and* for 2 additional days; show her how to prepare the solution.

- Explain to her how to continue the treatment of her child at home following Treatment Plan A.

Treatment of patients with severe dehydration — Treatment Plan C

Children with signs of *severe dehydration* can die quickly from hypovolaemic shock. They should be treated *immediately*, following Treatment Plan C (Fig. 5.3).

Tasks involved in Treatment Plan C

The main tasks of Treatment Plan C are:

- to decide how fluid will be given: (a) by intravenous drip, (b) by nasogastric infusion, or (c) orally;
- to decide how much intravenous fluid (or ORS solution) to give; then to give the fluid and reassess the patient frequently;
- to shift to Treatment Plan B or A when the child is no longer severely dehydrated;
- to treat suspected cases of cholera with an appropriate antimicrobial.

Deciding how fluid will be given

Intravenous replacement

The treatment of choice for severe dehydration is intravenous (IV) rehydration, because it is the most rapid way to restore the depleted blood volume. IV rehydration is

Fig. 5.3 **Treatment Plan C: for patients with severe dehydration**

TREATMENT PLAN C TO TREAT SEVERE DEHYDRATION QUICKLY

FOLLOW THE ARROWS. IF ANSWER IS "YES", GO ACROSS. IF "NO", GO DOWN

START HERE

Can you give intravenous (IV) fluids immediately?

YES →

- Start IV fluids immediately. If the patient can drink, give ORS by mouth while the drip is set up. Give 100 ml/kg Ringer's Lactate Solution (or, if not available, normal saline), divided as follows:

Age	First give 30 ml/kg in:	Then give 70 ml/kg in:
Infants (under 12 months)	1 hour *	5 hours
Older	30 minutes *	2 1/2 hours

* Repeat once if radial pulse is still very weak or not detectable.

- Reassess the patient every 1-2 hours. If hydration is not improving, give the IV drip more rapidly.
- Also give ORS (about 5 ml/kg/hour) as soon as the patient can drink: usually after 3-4 hours (infants) or 1-2 hours (older patients).
- After 6 hours (infants) or 3 hours (older patients), evaluate the patient using the assessment chart. Then choose the appropriate Plan (A, B or C) to continue treatment.

NO ↓

Is IV treatment available nearby, (within 30 minutes)?

YES →

- Send the patient immediately for IV treatment.
- If the patient can drink, provide the mother with ORS solution and show her how to give it during the trip.

NO ↓

Are you trained to use a naso-gastric (NG) tube for rehydration?

YES →

- Start rehydration by tube with ORS solution: Give 20 ml/kg/hour for 6 hours (total of 120 ml/kg).
- Reassess the patient every 1-2 hours:
  - If there is repeated vomiting or increasing abdominal distension, give the fluid more slowly.
  - If hydration is not improving after 3 hours, send the patient for IV therapy.
- After 6 hours, reassess the patient and choose the appropriate Treatment Plan.

NO ↓

Can the patient drink?

YES →

- Start rehydration by mouth with ORS solution, giving 20 ml/kg/hour for 6 hours (total of 120 ml/kg).
- Reassess the patient every 1-2 hours:
  - If there is repeated vomiting, give the fluid more slowly.
  - If hydration is not improving after 3 hours, send the patient for IV therapy.
- After 6 hours, reassess the patient and choose the appropriate Treatment Plan.

NO ↓

URGENT: Send the patient for IV or NG treatment

NOTES:

- If possible, observe the patient at least 6 hours after rehydration to be sure the mother can maintain hydration giving ORS solution by mouth.
- If the patient is above 2 years and there is cholera in your area, give an appropriate oral antibiotic after the patient is alert.

especially important if there are signs of hypovolaemic shock (i.e. the patient has a very rapid and weak, or absent radial pulse, cool and moist extremities, and is very lethargic or unconscious). Alternative routes for fluid replacement should only be used when IV rehydration is not possible or cannot be obtained nearby, within 30 minutes.

Nasogastric replacement

If IV therapy is not possible, a nasogastric (NG) tube can be used to give ORS solution, provided there is a person trained in its use. However, this approach is not as satisfactory as IV infusion because the fluid cannot be given as rapidly and additional time is required for it to be absorbed from the intestine. The maximum rate of fluid infusion is about 20 ml/kg per hour; with higher rates, abdominal distension and repeated vomiting are frequent problems.

Oral replacement

If IV and NG therapy are not possible, or will be delayed, and *the child is able to drink*, ORS solution should be given by mouth at a rate of 20 ml/kg per hour. This approach has the same disadvantages as NG therapy; moreover, it cannot be used for patients who are very lethargic or unconscious. Children under 2 years should be given ORS solution by spoon, about one teaspoonful per minute; older children and adults may take the solution from a cup. Patients with abdominal distension caused by paralytic ileus should not be given ORS solution either orally or by NG tube.

If fluid replacement is not possible by *any* of these routes, refer the child *urgently* to the nearest centre where IV or NG therapy can be given.

Intravenous rehydration

Selecting an appropriate intravenous fluid

A variety of different solutions is available for IV infusion (see Unit 2). However, some do not contain appropriate amounts of the electrolytes required to correct the deficits caused by diarrhoea. Ringer's lactate solution (also called Hartmann's solution for injection) is the preferred commercially available solution. If it is not available, normal saline (9 g NaCl/l), half-strength Darrow's solution with dextrose (25 g or 50 g/l) or half-normal saline with dextrose (50 g or 100 g/l) may be used. IV solutions containing only dextrose (glucose) should not be used.

Putting up an intravenous drip

IV therapy should be given only by trained persons. Some points to remember are given below (see also Annex 4):

- Needles, tubing, bottles, and fluid *must* be sterile.

- IV therapy can be given in any convenient vein. Those most suitable are in front of the elbow (antecubital vein) or, in infants, on the scalp. In cases of hypovolaemic shock, particularly in adults, simultaneous infusion into two veins may help to restore blood volume rapidly.

- When a peripheral vein cannot be found because of severe hypovolaemia, a needle may be introduced into the femoral vein where it must be held firmly in place. (The femoral vein is located just medial to the femoral artery, which can be easily identified by its pulsation.) A large amount of fluid can then be infused very rapidly. The infusion site should be changed to a peripheral vein as soon as one becomes evident. A venous incision ("cut-down") should not be necessary; this takes longer to perform and is liable to become infected.

- If IV therapy will be delayed and the patient is able to drink, start giving ORS solution by mouth until the drip is running.

Deciding how much intravenous fluid to give

If possible, patients should be weighed so that their fluid requirements can be determined accurately. The fluid deficit in severe dehydration equals 10% of body weight (i.e. 100 ml/kg).

Infants should be given IV fluid at a rate of 30 ml/kg in the first hour, followed by 70 ml/kg in the next 5 hours, thus providing a total of 100 ml/kg in 6 hours. *Older children and adults* should be given IV fluid at a rate of 30 ml/kg within 30 minutes, followed by 70 ml/kg in the next 2.5 hours, thus providing a total of 100 ml/kg in 3 hours. *For all patients* it is useful to mark the IV fluid bottle, indicating the level the fluid should reach after each hour of infusion.

After the first 30 ml/kg have been given, a strong radial pulse should be readily palpable. If it is still very weak and rapid, a second infusion of 30 ml/kg should be given at the same rate; however, this is rarely necessary. Small amounts of ORS solution should also be given by mouth (about 5 ml/kg per hour) as soon as the patient is able to drink, in order to provide additional potassium and base; this is usually possible after 3–4 hours for infants and 1–2 hours for older patients.

Reassessing the patient

During rehydration, the patient's progress should be assessed at least hourly until there is a definite improvement. Particular attention should be paid to:

- the signs of dehydration (see Fig. 3.1, page 34);
- the number and nature of the stools passed;
- any difficulty in giving fluids.

Signs of a satisfactory response to rehydration are: return of a strong radial pulse, improved level of consciousness, increased ability to drink, much improved skin turgor, and passage of urine. When these are seen, the interval between reassessments can be lengthened.

If the signs of dehydration remain unchanged or become worse, and especially if the patient has also passed several watery stools, the rate of fluid administration and the total amount given for rehydration should be increased.

Alternative methods of rehydration

Nasogastric rehydration

An NG tube (2.0–2.7 mm in diameter for a child, 4.0–6.0 mm for an adult) should be positioned by a person trained in its use (see Annex 5). While the tube is in place, the patient's head should be kept slightly raised to reduce the risk of regurgitated fluid entering the lungs.

Patients with severe dehydration should receive about 120 ml of ORS solution per kg of body weight over 6 hours, administered at a steady rate of 20 ml/kg per hr. This rate should be reduced only if there is repeated vomiting or increasing abdominal distension.

Patients should be reassessed every 1–2 hours until a satisfactory response to treatment is seen. If the signs of dehydration fail to improve or become worse after 3 hours of attempted NG rehydration, this approach is not likely to be successful and the patient should be sent urgently to a facility where IV treatment is possible.

Oral rehydration

The amount of fluid to be given orally and the monitoring of patients during oral rehydration are the same as described above for NG rehydration. It is helpful to measure out the amount of fluid required each hour into a glass or other container, even though it may be given by spoon. If a patient cannot drink the required amount of fluid or vomits frequently, the rate of administration should be slowed and the rehydration period lengthened. If signs of dehydration fail to improve or become worse after 3 hours of attempted oral rehydration, the patient should be sent urgently to a facility where IV treatment is possible.

Giving breast milk and water

Breast-feeding should be resumed as soon as an infant can suck. Infants less than 6 months of age who are not breast-fed should be given 100–200 ml of plain water during the first 6 hours, once they are able to drink; older children and adults should be given water to drink as soon as they desire it, provided that vomiting has subsided. (This is in addition to any ORS solution being given.)

Transition to Treatment Plans B and A

At the end of the planned rehydration period (usually 3–6 hours), the patient's hydration status should be carefully reassessed. If signs of severe dehydration are still present, rehydration therapy must be continued following Treatment Plan C. Otherwise, further treatment should follow Plan B or Plan A, depending, respectively, on whether signs of some dehydration remain or there are no signs of dehydration. In either case, ORS solution should be used and the patient should be given food and drink. Before removing the IV drip, it is wise to give ORS solution for at least 1 hour to be certain ORT is feasible. If possible, patients presenting with severe dehydration should stay in the health facility until the diarrhoea subsides. Otherwise, they should be observed for at least 6 hours after rehydration before returning home, to make sure that the mother can maintain their hydration using ORS solution.

Treatment of suspected cholera

Children over 2 years of age and adults with severe dehydration caused by acute watery diarrhoea, who live in an area where cholera is present, should be given an appropriate oral antimicrobial after vomiting subsides. This would usually be tetracycline, doxycycline or trimethoprim–sulfamethoxazole (see Annex 6). If *V. cholerae* O1 in the area are known to be resistant to these agents, furazolidone or chloramphenicol may be used. Treatment of cholera with an appropriate antimicrobial helps to shorten the duration of diarrhoea, but does not diminish the need for careful fluid replacement.

Possible complications

A number of problems may arise during rehydration therapy, some of which require specific treatment. In general, these fall into the three categories discussed below.

Electrolyte and acid–base abnormalities

These include hypernatraemia, hyponatraemia, hyperkalaemia, hypokalaemia, and base-deficit acidosis. The pathogenesis and clinical features of these disorders are described in Unit 2. Usually they arise as dehydration is developing or when the fluids used for rehydration do not have an appropriate composition. Although certain clinical features may suggest a particular diagnosis (e.g. seizures suggest hypernatraemia or hyponatraemia, and paralytic ileus suggests hypokalaemia), these signs are not specific and a diagnosis can be made with certainty only by measuring serum electrolytes, bicarbonate, or pH. It is important to understand, however, that these disorders are *all corrected* when ORS solution is used to treat dehydration as described in this unit and kidney function is normal.

Failure of oral rehydration therapy

A small number of patients with *some dehydration* cannot be treated adequately with ORS solution by mouth and require IV (or NG) therapy. They should receive Ringer's lactate solution (70 ml/kg intravenously over 3–4 hours) and then be reassessed to determine whether ORT is possible or IV treatment should be continued. Patients that fall into this category may have:

- *High rates of purging (frequent passage of voluminous liquid stools).* Patients who pass watery stools at very high rates (e.g. exceeding 15 ml/kg per hour) may be unable to drink sufficient ORS solution to replace their continuing stool losses, so that their signs of dehydration worsen. Such patients should be treated for several hours with IV fluid, until the rate of purging decreases.

- *Persistent vomiting.* Vomiting does not usually prevent successful ORT because most of the fluid taken is retained and absorbed, despite the obvious losses. When vomiting is frequent, the first step is to stop giving ORS solution for 10 minutes, and then to resume giving it, but more slowly; most patients can be managed successfully in this way. Occasionally, however, severe and repeated vomiting prevents effective oral rehydration. If the clinical signs of dehydration do not improve, or become worse, fluids should be given intravenously until the vomiting subsides. Remember that vomiting is often most severe during dehydration and usually disappears as water and electrolytes are replaced. Drugs should *never* be given to control vomiting because they are not very effective and often cause the child to become sleepy, making ORT more difficult.

- *Inability to drink.* Patients who cannot drink because of stomatitis (due, for example, to measles, *Candida*, or herpesvirus), fatigue, or central nervous system depression induced by drugs (such as antiemetics or antimotility drugs) should be given IV fluid or ORS solution by NG tube. If the patient is comatose, fluid should be given intravenously, if possible, or by NG tube.

- *Abdominal distension and paralytic ileus.* If the abdomen starts to become distended, ORS solution should be given more slowly. If abdominal distension continues to increase or is already well developed, and especially if there is paralytic ileus with absent bowel sounds, ORT or NG therapy should be stopped and fluid should be given intravenously. Paralytic ileus may be caused by opiate drugs (e.g. codeine, loperamide), hypokalaemia, or, more frequently, by both acting together.

- *Glucose malabsorption.* Clinically significant glucose malabsorption is unusual during acute diarrhoea. However, when it does occur, the use of ORS solution may cause a marked increase in watery diarrhoea with large amounts of unabsorbed glucose in the stool and worsening signs of dehydration (see Fig. 2.4, page 24). The child may also become hypernatraemic and very thirsty. Special tapes or test sticks can be used to detect glucose in the stool. Tests for reducing substances can also be used (see Unit 7). When glucose malabsorption prevents successful ORT, fluids should be given intravenously until diarrhoea subsides. Water may also be given to drink until thirst is satisfied.

Seizures

Dehydrated children occasionally develop convulsions either before or during rehydration therapy. Some possible causes of seizures and their appropriate treatment are as follows:

- *Hypoglycaemia.* This occurs mostly in malnourished infants and young children. A therapeutic test for hypoglycaemia in a comatose child involves giving sterile glucose solution (200 g/l) intravenously; if hypoglycaemia is the cause, giving 2.5 ml/kg of the solution over 5 minutes should cause a rapid improvement in consciousness. After waking up, the child should be fed and/or given ORS solution to prevent a recurrence.

- *Hyperthermia.* Some young children (especially infants) develop seizures when they have a fever; the risk is greatest when the fever is high, i.e. exceeds 40 °C. Treatment of high fever involves giving paracetamol, or cooling by sponging with tepid water and fanning.

- *Hypernatraemia or hyponatraemia.* See Unit 2 for a discussion of these conditions. The preferred treatment is with ORS solution, unless glucose malabsorption occurs

Fig. 5.4 **Correction of hypernatraemic or hyponatraemic dehydration in infants with ORS solution**

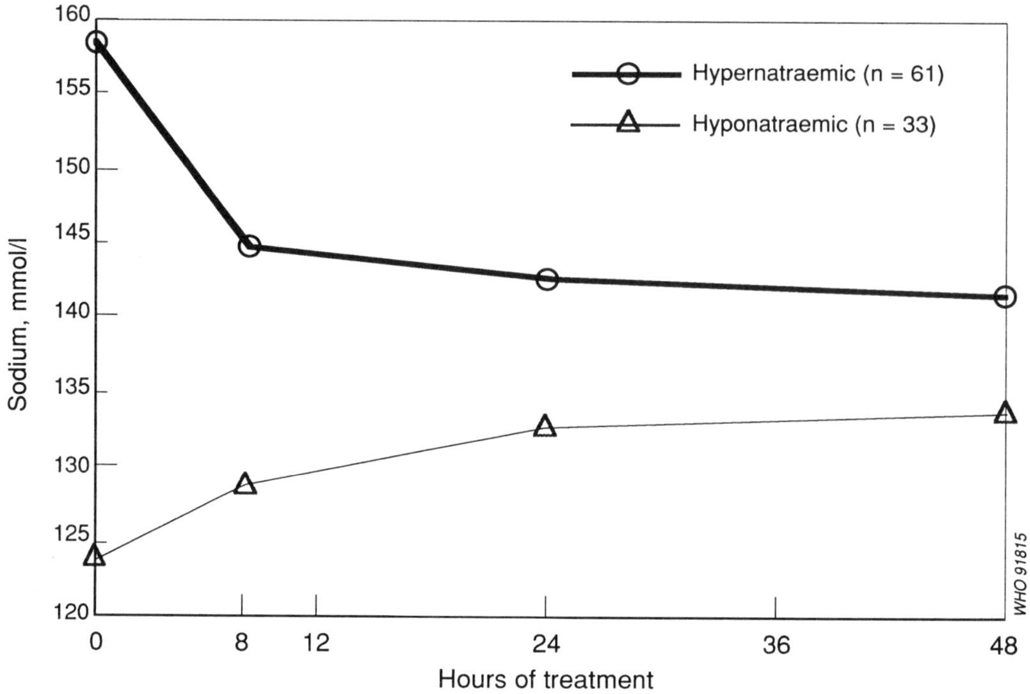

Source: Pizarro, D. et al. Oral dehydration in hypernatraemic and hyponatraemic diarrhoeal dehydration. *American journal of diseases of children*, **137**: 730–734 (1983).

(see page 75). When sufficient amounts are given to correct dehydration and restore normal kidney function, serum sodium levels will become normal within 24–48 hours and any modest excess of sodium or water is excreted in the urine. Fig. 5.4 shows how serum sodium concentration was corrected in infants who developed hypernatraemic or hyponatraemic dehydration owing to diarrhoea and were treated with ORS solution.

- *Central nervous system conditions unrelated to diarrhoea,* such as epilepsy or meningitis. Appropriate anticonvulsant and antimicrobial therapy should be given.

Exercises

1. Ahmed has diarrhoea and signs of some dehydration. He is 8 months old and weighs 6 kg. Approximately how much ORS solution should he be given during the first 4 hours of treatment? (Use the table in Fig. 5.1 to determine your answer.)

   A. 200–400 ml.
   B. 400–600 ml.
   C. 600–800 ml.
   D. 300–400 ml.

2. A mother has brought her 2-year-old daughter, Maria, to the health facility. Maria has been assessed and found to have signs of some dehydration. She weighs 12 kg.

While at the facility, her mother has given her 800 ml of ORS solution within 4 hours. After 4 hours, Maria still has signs of some dehydration, but is improving. Assuming that the mother can stay at the facility, what should be done next? (There may be more than one correct answer.)

A. Stop ORT and give 500 ml of Ringer's lactate solution intravenously during the next 3 hours.
B. Repeat Treatment Plan B, giving 800–1000 ml of ORS solution in the next 4 hours.
C. Pass an NG tube and give 900–1200 ml of ORS solution by this route in the next 4 hours.
D. Start to feed the child as described in Treatment Plan A.

3. John, an 18-month-old child with diarrhoea, has been brought to the health centre by his grandmother. He weighs 9 kg. He has been assessed and found to have signs of some dehydration. The grandmother must leave soon to catch the last bus; it is too far for her to walk home. What should the health worker do? (There may be more than one correct answer.)

A. Give the child an antimicrobial to treat his infection.
B. Give the grandmother 700 ml of ORS solution and show her how to give it to John during the next 4 hours.
C. Explain to the grandmother how John should be fed when they return home.
D. Give the grandmother two 1-litre packets of ORS for use in treating John at home during the next 2 days, after he has been rehydrated.

4. Balaji has been brought to a small health centre with signs of severe dehydration (he is very drowsy and cannot drink). He weighs 9 kg. There is no IV equipment at the health centre, but the health worker knows how to use an NG tube. How much ORS solution should be given through the NG tube in the first hour?

A. 30 ml/kg, i.e. 270 ml.
B. 20 ml/kg, i.e. 180 ml.
C. 10 ml/kg, i.e. 90 ml.
D. As much as possible, until abdominal distension occurs.

5. Omo is a 4-month-old baby weighing 4 kg who was severely dehydrated due to diarrhoea. He has received 250 ml of Ringer's lactate solution intravenously over 3 hours and is improving. He can now drink. What treatment should be given next? (There may be more than one correct answer.)

A. He should be treated according to Treatment Plan B.
B. He should resume breast-feeding.
C. He should receive 150 ml of Ringer's lactate solution intravenously in the next 3 hours.
D. He should begin taking small amounts of ORS solution, about 20 ml each hour.

6. Sanjay is a 3-month-old boy weighing 4 kg, who was severely dehydrated. He was given 400 ml of Ringer's lactate solution intravenously over 6 hours and is improving, but still has signs of some dehydration. What treatment should he receive now? (There may be more than one correct answer.)

A. He should be given 200–400 ml of ORS solution over the next 4 hours.
B. He should continue to receive IV treatment, following Treatment Plan C, until all signs of dehydration have disappeared.
C. He should be given an antidiarrhoeal drug or antimicrobial to help stop his diarrhoea.
D. His mother should resume breast-feeding him if she has not done so already.

7. You are a doctor working in an urban clinic. Ria, an 8-month-old girl, is brought to you. She is comatose, with a very rapid heart rate; you cannot feel her radial pulse; the skin of her arms and legs is cool and moist and her skin pinch goes back very slowly; her abdomen is distended and there are infrequent bowel sounds. Ria has been having profuse, watery diarrhoea and severe vomiting for the past 2 days. The local pharmacist prescribed antiemetic drops and a suspension containing codeine. The baby has a temperature of 38 °C and weighs 6 kg.

A. What type of dehydration does Ria have? ______________________
B. How much fluid is needed to replace her deficit? ______ ml
C. How should the fluid be given? ______________________
D. Over what time periods would you divide her rehydration therapy? ______
E. What is the probable cause of Ria's abdominal distension? ______________

8. Hawa has been brought to a local health facility. She is 3 years old and weighs 12 kg. She lives in an area where cholera has recently been diagnosed. Her diarrhoea started yesterday and she has passed six large watery stools. Her mother stopped giving her food, but started giving her extra liquids. However, Hawa has had severe vomiting all morning. As you examine her, you notice that she is very sleepy, has dry and very sunken eyes, and a very dry tongue; her skin pinch goes back very slowly. IV fluid is available at the health facility.

A. What type of dehydration does Hawa have? ______________________
B. You decide to give IV treatment, but Ringer's lactate solution is not available. What solution would be your next choice? ______________________
C. You suspect that Hawa may have cholera. What treatment should you give her? ______________________
D. When should you start to give Hawa ORS solution by mouth? ______________

9. Ali is 5 months old and weighs 4.5 kg. His mother breast-feeds him. His diarrhoea started last night, and he has passed eight very watery stools. His mother said there was no blood in the stools. As you examine Ali, you find that his skin pinch goes back slowly, his eyes are a little sunken, and he drinks some ORS solution very eagerly. Ali does not have a fever.

A. What type of dehydration does Ali have? ______________________
B. Which treatment plan should be followed for Ali? ______________________
C. Approximately how much ORS solution should Ali receive in the first 4 hours? ______ ml
D. When should the mother start to breast-feed Ali again? ______________
E. If Ali has no signs of dehydration after 4 hours, what treatment plan should be followed next? ______________________

UNIT 6

Dysentery, persistent diarrhoea, and diarrhoea associated with other illnesses

Introduction

For some children with diarrhoea, the combination of rehydration and diet therapy described in Treatment Plan A (see Unit 4) is not sufficient treatment. This applies in particular to children with dysentery or persistent diarrhoea, or whose illness is complicated by severe malnutrition or an infection outside the intestinal tract. While such patients may need rehydration, they may also require special approaches to feeding, antimicrobial therapy, or other treatment. This unit describes the management of children with dysentery, persistent diarrhoea, or other infections that may accompany or predispose to diarrhoea (see Fig. 6.1). The management of children with diarrhoea and severe malnutrition is considered in Unit 7.

Dysentery

Definition, etiology, and importance

Dysentery is defined as diarrhoea with visible blood in the stools. The most important and most frequent cause of acute dysentery is *Shigella*, especially *S. flexneri* and *S. dysenteriae* type 1. Other causes include *Campylobacter jejuni*, especially in infants, and, less frequently, *Salmonella;* dysentery caused by the latter agents is usually not severe. Enteroinvasive *Escherichia coli* is closely related to *Shigella* and may cause severe dysentery. However, infection with this agent is uncommon. *Entamoeba histolytica* causes dysentery in older children and adults, but rarely in children under 5 years of age.

Dysentery is an important cause of morbidity and mortality associated with diarrhoea. About 10% of all diarrhoeal episodes in children under 5 years are dysenteric, but these cause about 15% of all deaths attributed to diarrhoea. Dysentery is especially severe in infants and in children who are malnourished, develop clinically evident dehydration during their illness, or are not breast-fed. It also has a more harmful effect on nutritional status than acute watery diarrhoea. Dysentery occurs with increased frequency and severity in children who have measles or have had measles in the preceding month, and diarrhoeal episodes that begin with dysentery are more likely to become persistent than those that start with watery stools.

Clinical features and diagnosis

The clinical diagnosis of dysentery is based *solely* on the presence of visible blood in the diarrhoeal stool. The stool will also contain numerous pus cells (polymorphonuclear leukocytes) which are visible with a microscope, and it may contain large amounts of mucus; these latter features suggest infection with a bacterial agent that invades the intestinal mucosa (such as *Campylobacter jejuni* or *Shigella*), but alone are not sufficient to diagnose dysentery. In some episodes of shigellosis, the stool is initially watery, becoming bloody after 1 or 2 days. This watery diarrhoea is sometimes severe and may cause dehydration. Usually, however, numerous small bloody stools are passed and dehydration does not occur. Patients with dysentery frequently have fever, but sometimes the temperature is abnormally low, especially in the most serious cases. Cramping abdominal pain and pain in the rectum during defecation, or attempted defecation (tenesmus), are also common; however, young children are unable to describe these complaints.

Fig. 6.1 **Evaluation and management of patients with bloody diarrhoea, persistent diarrhoea, severe malnutrition or fever**

THEN, FOR OTHER PROBLEMS

ASK ABOUT BLOOD IN THE STOOL

IF BLOOD IS PRESENT:

- Treat for 5 days with an oral antibiotic recommended for **Shigella** in your area.
- Teach the mother to feed the child as described in Plan A.
- See the child again after 2 days if:
  - under 1 year of age
  - initially dehydrated
  - there is still blood in the stool
  - not getting better
- If the stool is still bloody after 2 days, change to a second oral antibiotic recommended for **Shigella** in your area. Give it for 5 days.

ASK WHEN THIS EPISODE OF DIARRHOEA BEGAN

IF DIARRHOEA HAS LASTED AT LEAST 14 DAYS:

- Refer to hospital if:
  - the child is under 6 months old
  - dehydration is present. (Refer the child after treatment of dehydration.)
- Otherwise, teach the mother to feed her child as in Plan A, except:
  - give only half the usual amount of milk, or replace milk with a fermented milk product, such as yoghurt.
  - assure full energy intake by giving 6 meals a day of thick cereal and added oil, mixed with vegetables, pulses, meat, or fish.
- Tell the mother to bring the child back after 5 days:
  - if diarrhoea has not stopped, refer to hospital.
  - if diarrhoea has stopped, tell the mother to:
    - use the same foods for the child's regular diet.
    - after 1 more week, gradually resume the usual animal milk.
    - give an extra meal each day for at least 1 month.

LOOK FOR SEVERE MALNUTRITION

IF THE CHILD HAS SEVERE MALNUTRITION:

- Do not attempt rehydration; refer to hospital for management.
- Provide the mother with ORS solution and show her how to give 5 ml/kg/hr during the trip.

ASK ABOUT FEVER AND TAKE TEMPERATURE

IF THE CHILD IS UNDER 2 MONTHS OF AGE:

- Rehydrate as necessary. If there is fever (38° C or above) after rehydration, refer to hospital. Do not give paracetamol or an antimalarial.

IF THE CHILD IS 2 MONTHS OF AGE OR OLDER:

- If temperature is 39° C or above, give paracetamol.
- If there is falciparum malaria in the area, and the child has any fever (38° C or above) or history of fever in the past 5 days, give an antimalarial (or manage according to your malaria programme recommendation).

A number of severe and potentially fatal complications can occur during dysentery, especially when the cause is *Shigella*. They include intestinal perforation, toxic megacolon, rectal prolapse, convulsions (with or without a high fever), septicaemia, haemolytic–uraemic syndrome, and prolonged hyponatraemia. A major complication of dysentery is weight loss and rapid worsening of nutritional status. This is caused by anorexia (which may be marked), the body's increased need for nutrients to fight infection and repair damaged tissue, and the loss of serum protein from the damaged intestine (i.e. protein-losing enteropathy). Death from dysentery is usually caused by extensive damage to the ileum and colon, complications of sepsis, secondary infection (e.g. pneumonia), or severe malnutrition. Children convalescing from dysentery are also at increased risk of death from other infections, owing perhaps to their poor nutritional state or impaired immunity.

The cause of an episode of dysentery often goes undetermined. Stool culture, to detect pathogenic bacteria, is often impossible. Moreover, at least 2 days are required before results of a culture are available, whereas a decision on antimicrobial therapy must be made immediately. Stool microscopy to detect protozoa may also be unavailable or unreliable. Amoebiasis can only be diagnosed with certainty when trophozoites of *E. histolytica* containing red blood cells are seen in fresh stools or in mucus from rectal ulcers (obtained during proctoscopy). The detection of cysts alone is *not* sufficient for a diagnosis of amoebiasis. Amoebiasis should be suspected when a child with dysentery does not improve following appropriate antimicrobial therapy for shigellosis.

Management

Children with dysentery should be presumed to have shigellosis and treated accordingly. This is because shigellae cause about 60% of dysentery cases seen at health facilities and nearly all cases of severe, life-threatening disease. If microscopic examination of the stool is performed and trophozoites of *E. histolytica* containing erythrocytes are seen, antiamoebic therapy should also be given (see below). The four key components of the treatment of dysentery (see Fig. 6.1) are:

- antimicrobials;
- fluids;
- feeding;
- follow-up.

Antimicrobial therapy

Early treatment of shigellosis with an appropriate antimicrobial shortens the duration of the illness and reduces the risk of serious complications and death; however, such treatment is effective only when the shigellae are sensitive to the antimicrobial that is given. If treatment is delayed or an antimicrobial is given to which the shigellae are not sensitive, the bacteria may cause extensive damage to the bowel and enter the general circulation, causing septicaemia, prostration, and sometimes septic shock. These complications occur more frequently in children who are malnourished or in infants, and may be fatal.

Since the antimicrobial sensitivity of the infecting strain of *Shigella* is not known for each case, it is important to use an oral antimicrobial to which most shigellae in the area are known to be sensitive. Trimethoprim–sulfamethoxazole is the usual choice, but ampicillin is effective in some areas (see Annex 6). Although treatment is recommended for 5 days, there should be a substantial improvement after 2 days, i.e. reduced fever, less pain and faecal blood, and fewer loose stools. If this does not occur, the antimicrobial should be stopped and a different one used; in many areas this would be nalidixic acid. Although other bacteria, such as *Campylobacter jejuni* and *Salmonella,* can cause dysentery, the disease is usually relatively mild and self-limiting.

Young children with dysentery should *not* be treated routinely for amoebiasis. Treatment should be given only when *E. histolytica* trophozoites containing red blood cells are identified in faeces or when bloody stools persist after consecutive treatment with two antimicrobials (each given for 2 days) that are usually effective for *Shigella*. The preferred treatment for amoebic dysentery is metronidazole (see Annex 6). If dysentery is caused by *E. histolytica*, an improvement will occur within 2–3 days of starting treatment.

Fluids

Children with dysentery should be evaluated for signs of dehydration and treated accordingly (see Units 3–5). All patients with dysentery should be offered water and other recommended fluids during their illness, especially if they have fever.

Feeding

Children with dysentery should continue to be fed in order to prevent or minimize nutritional damage. Feeding may be difficult, however, because of anorexia. The general feeding guidelines in Treatment Plan A (Units 4 and 7) should be followed.

Follow-up

Most patients with dysentery show substantial improvement within 2 days after beginning treatment with an effective antimicrobial. These patients should complete the 5-day treatment, and do not usually require follow-up. Other patients should be followed closely, particularly children who do not show a clear improvement within 2 days, and children known to be at high risk of death or other complications. High-risk children (i.e. infants, malnourished children, those not breast-fed, and any who have been dehydrated) should be monitored frequently as outpatients or admitted to hospital. Patients with dysentery and severe malnutrition should be admitted to hospital routinely. Children showing no improvement after the first 2 days of antimicrobial treatment should be given a different antimicrobial, as described above.

Prevention

The microorganisms that cause dysentery are spread by faecally contaminated hands, food, and water. The spread of shigellosis by hands is very efficient because the number of shigellae required to cause disease is very small (as few as 10–100 organisms). Important measures to prevent shigellosis include careful hand-washing and use of latrines; these are described in Unit 8.

Persistent diarrhoea

Definition, etiology, and importance

Persistent diarrhoea is a diarrhoeal episode that lasts for 14 days or longer (see Unit 1). About 10% of acute diarrhoeal episodes become persistent. Persistent diarrhoea often causes nutritional status to deteriorate and is associated with increased mortality. It causes about 35% of all diarrhoea-associated deaths, and as many as 15% of episodes of persistent diarrhoea result in death. There is no single microbial cause, although *Shigella, Salmonella* and enteroaggregative *E. coli* probably play a greater role than other agents; *Cryptosporidium* may also be important in severely malnourished or immunodeficient patients. A number of other pathogenic bacteria and protozoa are found with nearly equal frequency in cases of acute and persistent diarrhoea, but their role in the etiology of this disease is unclear. Irrespective of its cause, persistent diarrhoea is associated with extensive changes in the bowel mucosa, especially flattening of the villi and reduced production of disaccharidase enzymes; these cause reduced absorption of nutrients and may perpetuate the illness after the original infectious cause has been eliminated.

Risk factors

A number of risk factors for persistent diarrhoea have been identified:

- *Malnutrition* — this delays the repair of damaged intestinal epithelium, causing diarrhoea to be prolonged.
- *Recent introduction of animal milk or formula* — this could reflect lactose intolerance, hypersensitivity to milk protein, bacterial contamination of the milk, or some other mechanism. Animal milk appears to be an important factor in 30–40% of episodes of persistent diarrhoea.
- *Young age* — most episodes occur in children under 18 months of age.
- *Immunological impairment* — this is seen in severely malnourished children, during or following measles or some other viral infections, and in patients with the acquired immunodeficiency syndrome (AIDS).
- *Recent diarrhoea* — this includes children who have experienced a recent episode of acute diarrhoea or a previous episode of persistent diarrhoea.

Knowledge of these risk factors helps to identify children who are most likely to develop persistent diarrhoea and, in some instances, to guide treatment.

Nutritional impact

Persistent diarrhoea is largely a nutritional disease. It occurs more frequently in children who are already malnourished and is itself an important cause of malnutrition. A single episode of persistent diarrhoea can last 3–4 weeks or longer and cause dramatic weight loss, sometimes leading rapidly to severe malnutrition, i.e. marasmus.

Weight loss during persistent diarrhoea is caused by reduced absorption of all nutrients, but especially of fat and, in some children, lactose. Other contributing factors include poor food intake, owing to anorexia or withholding of food, or giving dilute, low-energy foods. Patients are also likely to be deficient in various vitamins and minerals: those of particular importance because of their role in the renewal and repair of the intestinal mucosa and/or their role in normal immunological responses include folate, vitamin B_{12}, vitamin A, zinc and iron.

Management

The initial management of children with persistent diarrhoea is summarized in Fig. 6.1 and discussed below.

History and examination

These should cover the same areas as in cases of acute diarrhoea, but with special attention to the following questions:

- How many days has this episode of diarrhoea lasted?
- What is the child being fed, breast milk or animal milk? If over 4–6 months of age, are the type and amount of weaning food adequate? How many meals are given each day? How is the child's appetite?
- Was animal milk or formula introduced recently? Does the diarrhoea seem to be worse soon after animal milk or formula is given?
- Is blood present in the stool?
- If this is a repeat visit, has the mother noted any change since the last visit in frequency of diarrhoea, blood in the stool, or the child's appetite? Could she follow the advice given at that time about treating the child?
- Is the child dehydrated?
- What is the child's nutritional status? Has it declined during this illness? Measure and plot weight-for-age (and weight-for-height, if possible).

Laboratory studies

For all patients, it is important to observe whether the stool is bloody. The use of other laboratory examinations will depend upon their availability. Some of the most useful ones are summarized in Table 6.1.

Fluid and electrolyte replacement

The child's hydration status should be assessed as described in Unit 3. ORS solution is satisfactory for replacing losses of water and salts in most children with persistent diarrhoea; a few patients have severe glucose malabsorption (see Unit 5) and require intravenous fluid therapy. Some patients with persistent diarrhoea develop dehydration and continue to pass stools rapidly after rehydration; they should be admitted to

Table 6.1 **Laboratory examinations in persistent diarrhoea**

Examination	What the examination will reveal
Observation of stool	Blood suggests infection with *Shigella*.
Stool microscopy	Red blood cells or white blood cells (polymorphonuclear leukocytes) suggest an invasive bacterial infection, such as shigellosis. Cysts or trophozoites of *Giardia,* or trophozoites of *E. histolytica*, suggest they may play a role in the disease.
Stool culture and sensitivity	Bacterial pathogens are detected and their antimicrobial sensitivity determined.
Stool pH, reducing substances	Stool pH of less than 5.5 and a large amount of reducing substances in the faeces indicate carbohydrate (most likely lactose) malabsorption. These findings do not mean, however, that this is necessarily the cause of the diarrhoea (see Unit 7).

hospital and may require treatment with intravenous fluids until the rate of purging declines.

Nutritional therapy

Proper feeding is the most important aspect of treatment for most children with persistent diarrhoea. Many can be treated on an outpatient basis with food available in the home; however, some require specialized care in hospital. Weight gain provides the best evidence that dietary management is effective, even before diarrhoea stops. The goals of nutritional therapy are:

- to reduce temporarily the amount of animal milk (or lactose) in the diet;
- to provide a sufficient intake of energy, protein, vitamins, and minerals to facilitate the repair process in the damaged gut mucosa and improve nutritional status;
- to avoid giving foods or drinks that may aggravate the diarrhoea;
- to ensure that the child's food intake during convalescence is adequate to correct any malnutrition.

The general guidelines for feeding during and after diarrhoea given in Treatment Plan A (see Unit 4) should be followed. Some important exceptions and additional guidelines are shown in Fig. 6.1 and given below.

- Children under 6 months of age or with evidence of dehydration should be rehydrated and referred to hospital for further management. They may require special measures to maintain hydration, replacement of animal milk with lactose-free or milk-free formula, special diets, laboratory studies to identify pathogenic bacteria or protozoa in their faeces, or other specialized procedures.

- For older children, the mother should be instructed to:

  —continue breast-feeding;
  —give only half the usual amount of animal milk or replace it with a fermented milk product, such as yoghurt. This reduces by half the amount of lactose in the child's diet. In many cases, this step will cause the diarrhoea to subside rapidly;

—ensure a *full energy intake* for the child (i.e. about 110 kcal/kg per day) by giving thick cereal with added vegetable oil; mix this with other foods, such as well-cooked and mashed pulses, vegetables, and if possible, finely ground chicken or fish. Avoid low-energy foods that are dilute or bulky. At least half of the child's energy intake should come from foods other than milk or milk products;
—avoid foods that are hyperosmolar (these are usually foods or drinks made very sweet by the addition of sucrose, such as soft drinks or commercial fruit drinks); these can make the diarrhoea worse;
—give food in frequent small meals, at least six times a day;
—provide supplementary vitamins and minerals, in particular folate, vitamin B_{12}, vitamin A, zinc and iron, if possible.

- Tell the mother to follow these instructions for 5 days and then bring the child back to be checked:

—if the diarrhoea has not stopped, refer the child to hospital for specialized care;
—if the diarrhoea has stopped, tell the mother to:

- continue to give the same foods for one more week;
- then, gradually reintroduce the usual animal milk or formula (if the child normally takes it) over several days and shift to a full-strength diet appropriate for the child's age;
- give an extra meal each day for at least 1 month. If the child is malnourished, this regimen should be continued until the deficit of weight-for-height is corrected. The child should be seen at monthly intervals to monitor growth (see Annex 3) and ensure that the feeding guidelines are being followed.

Drug therapy

Patients with persistent diarrhoea and blood in the stool or a stool culture positive for *Shigella* should receive an antimicrobial for shigellosis. If stool culture yields another bacterial pathogen, e.g. enteropathogenic *E. coli,* an oral antimicrobial to which that agent is sensitive should be given. If *Giardia* cysts, or trophozoites of either *Giardia* or *E. histolytica* are seen in the faeces or small bowel fluid, a course of appropriate antiprotozoal therapy should be given (see Annex 6). However, "blind" therapy with antimicrobials or antiprotozoal agents is *not* effective and should *not* be given; such treatment may make the illness worse. Similarly, no "antidiarrhoeal" drug (including antimotility drugs, antisecretory drugs and adsorbents) has any proven value in patients with persistent diarrhoea; such drugs should *not* be given (see also Unit 4).

Diarrhoea associated with other illnesses

Children with diarrhoea may also have other potentially serious illnesses, especially malnutrition or other infections. Two nutritional disorders associated with diarrhoea are considered in Units 3 and 7: vitamin A deficiency and severe malnutrition. The following discussion concerns infections that may be associated with diarrhoea.

Measles-associated diarrhoea

The incidence of diarrhoea is increased during measles, during the 4 weeks following the illness, and possibly for up to 6 months after the measles episode. Measles-associated diarrhoea is often severe and of longer than usual duration; the risk of death is also substantially higher than with diarrhoea that is not related to measles, and is probably even greater when children are also malnourished. Where the incidence of measles is high, measles-associated diarrhoea can account for one-third or more of diarrhoea-associated deaths in young children. Immunization against measles is therefore an important measure for preventing both diarrhoeal episodes and diarrhoea-associated deaths, as well as for preventing measles (see Unit 8).

The mechanisms by which measles predisposes to diarrhoea are not clear but may include: (i) a direct effect of measles virus on the bowel epithelium, and (ii) virus-induced immunosuppression, which can last for several months after an episode of measles and reduces the child's defences against a variety of pathogenic bacteria and protozoa. Patients with measles-associated diarrhoea frequently pass blood in the stool, suggesting that *Shigella* is an important causative agent.

The evaluation of children with diarrhoea should include an enquiry about recent measles. Treatment of measles-associated diarrhoea should include:

- treatment of dehydration and dysentery, when present;
- adequate feeding (as described in Treatment Plan A, Fig. 4.1, page 50);
- oral care for patients with stomatitis, so that this does not interfere with eating;
- administration of a prophylactic dose of vitamin A (see Unit 7).

Pneumonia and diarrhoea

Diarrhoea with severe dehydration causes rapid breathing that may suggest a diagnosis of pneumonia. However, in pneumonia the respiratory rate equals or exceeds 40 breaths per minute (50 breaths per minute for infants aged 2–11 months), the child is coughing, and subcostal chest indrawing may be seen. In children with severe dehydration, the breathing pattern improves rapidly when dehydration is corrected. If pneumonia is confirmed, an appropriate antimicrobial should be given.

Fever and diarrhoea

Fever is frequent in patients with diarrhoea. It is often present when diarrhoea is caused by rotavirus or an invasive bacterium such as *Shigella, Campylobacter jejuni* or *Salmonella*. Fever may also accompany dehydration and disappear during rehydration.

Fever in a patient with diarrhoea may also be a sign of another infection such as pneumonia, otitis media, or malaria. Patients with diarrhoea and fever should be examined for other infections and treated appropriately. However, it is *not* appropriate to give antimicrobials to patients with diarrhoea simply because they have fever. A more specific indication is required, such as pneumonia or bloody stools. If one is not found, the patient should be observed, and the search for the cause of the fever continued, if it persists.

Children 2 months of age or older, who have fever (38 °C or above) or a history of fever during the past 5 days and who live in an area where there is falciparum malaria, should be given an antimalarial or managed according to the recommendations of the national malaria control programme (see Fig. 6.1). If the child's temperature is 39 °C or greater, the child should be treated to reduce it. This may be done by giving paracetamol or, when fever is very high, by also sponging the head and abdomen with tepid water and fanning.

Infants less than 2 months of age, who have a temperature of 38 °C or above, should be treated for severe dehydration, if present, and then referred to hospital. Paracetamol or antimalarial drugs should not be given before referral.

Exercises

1. Ayaz, who is 2 years old, is brought to the health centre because he has had diarrhoea with blood in the stool for 3 days. The health worker assesses Ayaz and finds that he has no signs of dehydration and is neither febrile nor malnourished. What should the health worker do? (There may be more than one correct answer.)

   A. Treat Ayaz with metronidazole for possible amoebiasis, since he has no fever.
   B. Refer Ayaz to the nearest hospital for a stool examination and culture.
   C. Advise the mother to continue feeding Ayaz a nutrient-rich diet.
   D. Treat Ayaz for 5 days with an antimicrobial effective for *Shigella* in the area.
   E. Advise the mother to bring Ayaz back if blood has not disappeared from the stool after 2 days of treatment.

2. Pedro is 9 months old. He was well until 3 months ago when his mother stopped breast-feeding and began giving him cow's milk with other food. Since then Pedro has had three episodes of diarrhoea, the current one having begun 18 days ago. Pedro still takes cow's milk but his mother has reduced his intake of solid food since the diarrhoea began. There has been no blood in the stool. Pedro weighs 6 kg. What should the health worker do?

   A. Prescribe a special lactose-free formula and advise the mother to give this in place of the cow's milk.
   B. Give Pedro metronidazole for possible giardiasis.
   C. Advise the mother to give Pedro half the usual amount of milk each day and to increase other energy-rich foods in his diet, e.g. by adding some vegetable oil to his cooked cereal.
   D. Tell the mother to give Pedro sweetened fruit drinks or soft drinks, which he likes, so that he receives enough fluid.
   E. Tell the mother to bring Pedro back in 5 days.

3. Maria, aged 16 months, began having watery diarrhoea. After 2 days, her mother noted some blood in the stool and brought her to the health centre. The doctor

noted that Maria had a fever (39 °C) and saw that the stool contained blood. There was no evidence of malnutrition. The doctor gave her trimethoprim–sulfamethoxazole, but her mother came back after 2 days saying Maria had not improved and the stool was still bloody. What should the doctor do next?

A. Tell the mother to continue giving Maria trimethoprim–sulfamethoxazole, since it is supposed to be given for 5 days and she has given it for only 2 days.
B. Send Maria to the hospital for a stool culture.
C. Treat Maria with metronidazole for possible amoebiasis.
D. Stop the trimethoprim–sulfamethoxazole and give another antimicrobial to which most *Shigella* in the area are sensitive, e.g. nalidixic acid.
E. Treat Maria with erythromycin for a possible infection with *Campylobacter jejuni.*

4. Alam is 7 months old and takes only formula milk. He has had watery diarrhoea for the past 14 days. During the illness, Alam has continued to take his formula. He has not had a fever. How should he be treated? (There may be more than one correct answer.)

   A. Alam should be given an antiprotozoal agent effective for *Giardia.*
   B. Alam's mother should give him only half the usual amount of formula milk each day. She should also give him cooked cereal with oil and some well-cooked vegetables to ensure an adequate intake of nutrients. If the diarrhoea has not stopped in 5 days, he should be referred to hospital for further evaluation and treatment.
   C. Alam should be referred to hospital for special dietary care. This may require replacement of his usual milk with a lactose-free or soya-based formula.
   D. Alam's stool should be cultured and examined for *E. histolytica* and *Giardia.*
   E. Alam should receive an antidiarrhoeal drug to help control the diarrhoea.

5. Chinta is 14 months old. She has had a fever and watery diarrhoea for 3 days. Today some blood was seen in the stool. When seen in the health centre, she is well nourished, drinks ORS eagerly, and has reduced skin turgor. Chinta lives in an area where falciparum malaria occurs. Which of the following steps are appropriate? (There may be more than one correct answer.)

   A. Chinta should be given an antimalarial effective for falciparum malaria or managed according to the recommendations of the national malaria control programme.
   B. Chinta should receive oral rehydration following Treatment Plan B for *some dehydration.*
   C. Chinta should receive treatment for shigellosis, using an antimicrobial to which *Shigella* in the area are usually sensitive.
   D. Chinta's mother should continue to give her a normal nutrient-rich diet, feeding her frequent small meals.
   E. Chinta's mother should bring her back after 2 days of treatment to be certain she is responding adequately.

UNIT 7
Diarrhoea and nutrition

Interaction of diarrhoea and malnutrition

Diarrhoea is an important cause of malnutrition. This is because nutrient requirements are increased during diarrhoea, as during other infectious diseases, whereas nutrient intake and absorption are usually decreased. Each episode of diarrhoea can cause weight loss and growth faltering. Moreover, if diarrhoea occurs frequently, there may be too little time to "catch up" on growth (i.e. to make up for the growth that failed to occur) between episodes. The result can be a flattening of the normal growth curve, as shown in Fig. 7.1. Children who experience frequent episodes of acute diarrhoea, or have persistent diarrhoea, are more likely to become malnourished than children who experience fewer or shorter episodes of diarrhoea. In general, the impact of diarrhoea on nutritional status is proportional to the number of days a child spends with diarrhoea each year.

Fig. 7.1 **Growth pattern of a child with frequent episodes of diarrhoea and other infections**

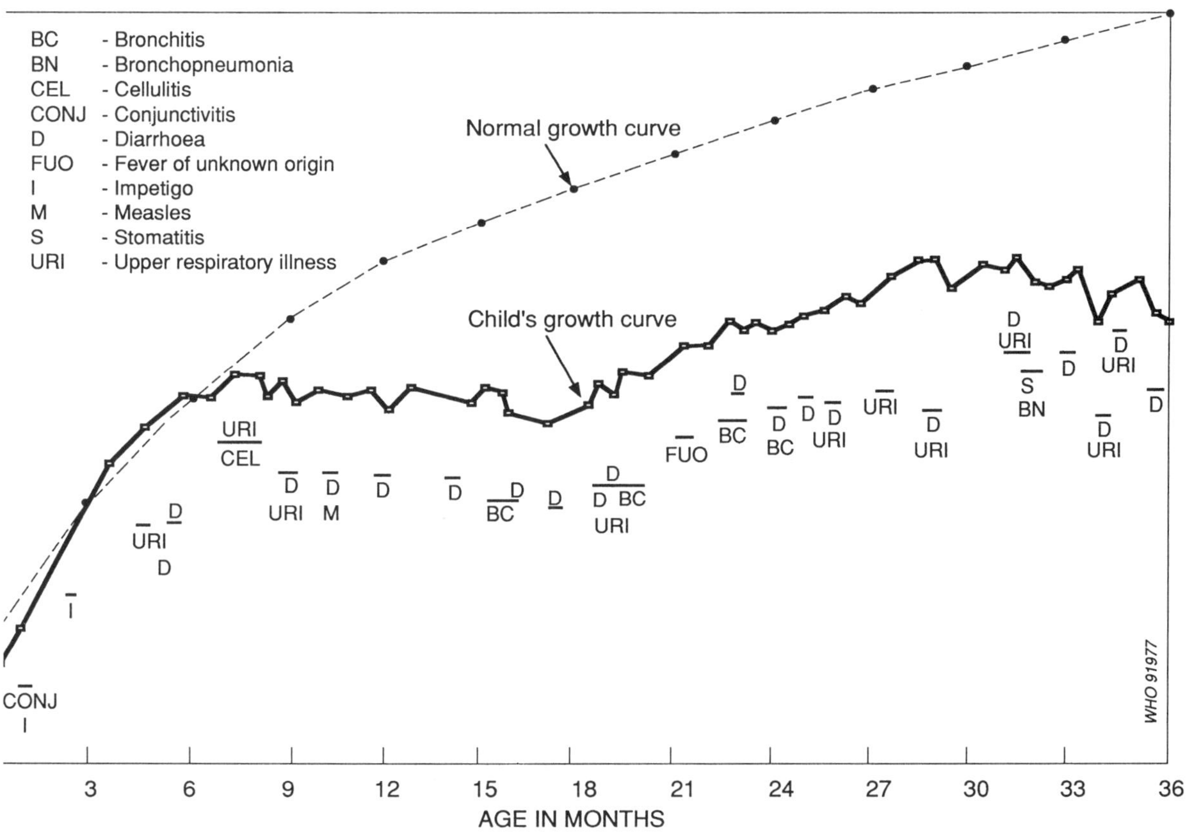

Source: Mata, L.J. Nutrition and infection. *Protein Advisory Group bulletin,* **11**: 18–21 (1971).

Malnutrition also contributes substantially to the problem of diarrhoea. In children who are malnourished as a result of inadequate feeding, acute diarrhoeal episodes are more severe, longer lasting, and possibly more frequent; persistent diarrhoea is also more frequent and dysentery is more severe. The risk of dying from an episode of persistent diarrhoea or dysentery is considerably increased when a child is already malnourished. In general, these effects are proportional to the degree of malnutrition, being greatest when malnutrition is severe.

Fig. 7.2 **Interaction of diarrhoea and malnutrition**

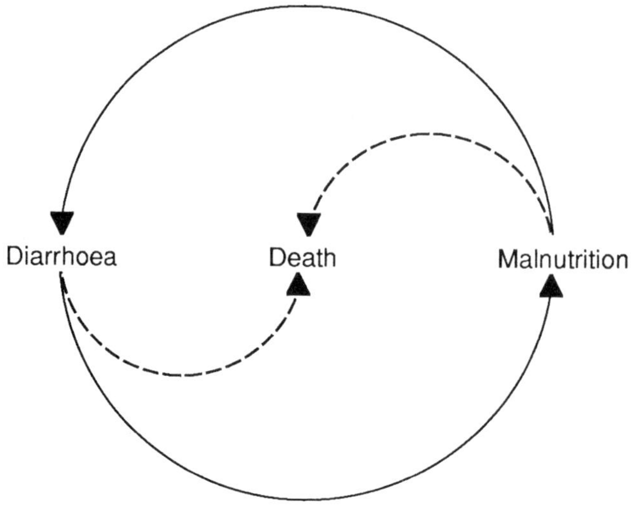

Thus, diarrhoea and malnutrition combine to form a vicious circle (Fig. 7.2) which, if it is not broken, can eventually result in death; the final event may be a particularly severe or prolonged episode of diarrhoea or, when severe malnutrition is present, another serious infection such as pneumonia. Deaths from diarrhoea are, in fact, usually associated with malnutrition. In hospitals where good management of dehydration is practised, virtually all deaths due to diarrhoea occur in malnourished children.

Diarrhoea is, in reality, as much a nutritional disease as one of fluid and electrolyte imbalance, and therapy is not adequate unless both aspects of the disease are treated. However, in contrast to fluid replacement, nutritional management of diarrhoea requires good feeding practices both during the illness and between episodes of diarrhoea, when the child is not sick. When this is done, and malnutrition is either prevented or corrected, the risk of death from a future episode of diarrhoea is greatly reduced.

This unit describes the factors responsible for nutritional decline during diarrhoea and considers how this effect can be reversed, and nutritional status maintained or improved, by appropriate feeding during and after an episode of diarrhoea.

Causes of nutritional decline during diarrhoea

Reduced food intake

Nutrient intake may decline by 30% or more during the first few days of acute diarrhoea as a result of:

- anorexia, which is especially marked in children with dysentery;
- vomiting, which discourages attempts at feeding;
- withholding of food, based on traditional beliefs about the treatment of diarrhoea or on recommendations by health personnel to "rest the bowel";

- giving foods with reduced nutrient value, such as gruel or soup that is diluted; this may be done in the belief that a diluted food is easier to digest.

Decreased absorption of nutrients

Overall nutrient absorption is also reduced by about 30% during acute diarrhoea, the impairment being greater for fats and proteins than for carbohydrates. Greater impairment can occur in malnourished children with persistent diarrhoea, reflecting more extensive damage to the gut mucosa. Decreased absorption of nutrients is caused by:

- damage to the absorptive (villous) epithelial cells, which reduces the total absorptive surface of the bowel;
- disaccharidase deficiency, owing to impaired production of enzymes by the damaged microvilli (when severe, this can cause malabsorption of disaccharide sugars, particularly lactose);
- reduced intestinal concentrations of bile acids, which are required for absorption of fats;
- rapid transit of food through the gut, leaving insufficient time for digestion and absorption.

Increased nutrient requirements

Nutrient requirements are increased during diarrhoea owing to:

- the metabolic demands associated with fever;
- the need to repair the damaged gut epithelium;
- the need to replace serum protein lost through the damaged intestinal mucosa, as occurs in dysentery.

Effects of feeding during and after diarrhoea

To prevent growth faltering, good nutrition must be maintained both during and after an episode of diarrhoea. This can be achieved by continuing to give generous amounts of nutritious foods throughout the episode and during convalescence. *In general, the foods that should be given during diarrhoea are the same as those the child should receive when he or she is well.* This approach is based on evidence that, during diarrhoea, the major proportion of most nutrients is digested, absorbed, and used, and that, during convalescence, substantial recovery of lost growth is possible. The effects of feeding on both the diarrhoeal illness and the child's nutritional status are considered below.

Effect of feeding on diarrhoea

The notion that feeding should be reduced or stopped during diarrhoea reflects a common belief that giving food will cause stool output to increase and thus make the diarrhoea worse, but this is not usually the case. For example:

- Breast milk is usually well tolerated during diarrhoea; children who continue to breast-feed during diarrhoea actually have reduced stool output and a shorter duration of illness than children who do not breast-feed.

- Feeding hastens repair of the intestinal mucosa, and stimulates early recovery of pancreatic function and production of brush-border disaccharidase enzymes. This leads to earlier return of normal digestion and improved absorption of nutrients.

- Children on mixed diets, e.g. cow's milk, cooked cereal, and vegetables, do not have increased stool output. However, those taking *only* animal milk or formula may have some increase in stool volume.

Food is usually well tolerated during diarrhoea, the major exception being clinically significant intolerance of lactose, and occasionally of protein in animal milk. This is unusual in acute diarrhoea, but can be a significant problem in children with persistent diarrhoea (see page 101 and Unit 6).

Effect of feeding on nutritional status

Food given during diarrhoea

A substantial proportion of food given during diarrhoea is digested and absorbed. It is not surprising, therefore, that children given full-strength feedings throughout an episode of diarrhoea gain weight at a near-normal rate, whereas those with a reduced intake gain much less or actually lose weight. Fig. 7.3 shows the growth pattern of

Fig. 7.3 **Effect of feeding on weight gain during diarrhoea**

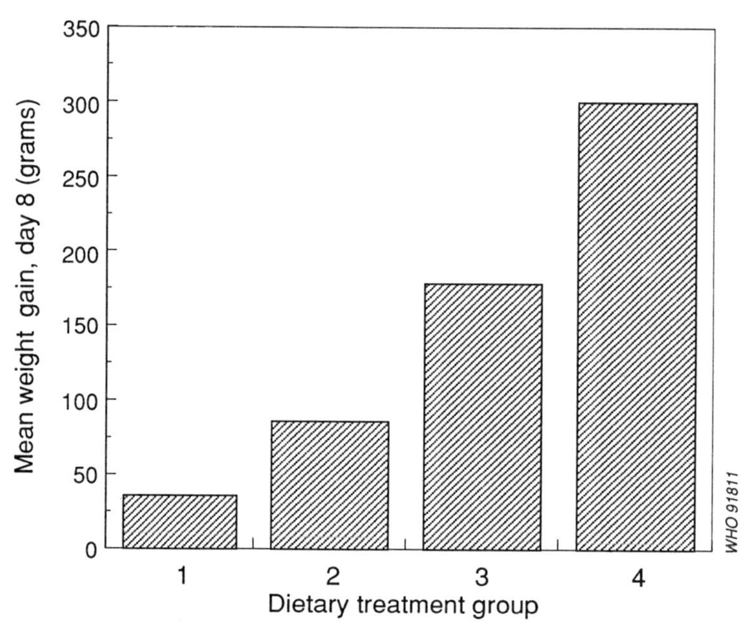

Day	Dietary intake (kcal/kg) on indicated day			
1-2	IV fluid	ORS	55	110
3-4	55	55	110	110
5-6	110	110	110	110

Source: Brown, K.H. et al. Effect of continued feeding on clinical and nutritional outcomes of acute diarrhoea in children. *Journal of pediatrics*, **112**: 191–200 (1988).

children given either a reduced or a full caloric intake during the first 4 days of an acute episode of diarrhoea. The figure shows that weight gain 8 days after starting treatment was greatest in those who received a normal caloric intake (110 kcal/kg per day) throughout their illness, and less in those whose food was reduced (55 kcal/kg per day) or withheld during the first 2–4 days of treatment. Moreover, there was no appreciable difference in the amount of diarrhoeal stool passed when children were fed half-strength or full-strength diets. On the basis of studies such as this, it is now clear that *there is no evidence to support a reduction in food intake during diarrhoea.* Instead, full-strength feeding should be continued so that growth faltering and worsening of nutritional status can be prevented, or at least minimized.

Food given after diarrhoea stops

Even when a child is given as much food as possible during diarrhoea, some growth faltering may occur, especially if the child has marked anorexia. Moreover, many children are malnourished prior to developing diarrhoea and will remain at increased risk of frequent, severe, or prolonged episodes of diarrhoea until their nutritional status improves. The goal of feeding after diarrhoea stops is to correct malnutrition and to achieve and sustain a normal pattern of growth. This is best done by ensuring that the child's *normal diet* provides enough energy and other required nutrients. This is most important for children older than 4–6 months of age receiving a mixed diet. The foods recommended for such children during diarrhoea (see below) are those recommended for normal feeding when the child is well. It is also helpful to give increased amounts of nutrient-rich food during the first few weeks of convalescence, when children are often very hungry and may readily consume 50% or even 100% more calories than usual and grow at several times their normal rate.

Nutritional management of diarrhoea

The vicious circle by which diarrhoea and malnutrition interact can be broken by correct feeding practices. This requires that health workers advise mothers on the best way to feed their children normally, teach them the importance of continued, full-strength feeding during diarrhoea, and assist them in their efforts to follow this advice. The four key components of correct nutritional management of diarrhoea in children are:

- assessing the nutritional status of the child;
- appropriate feeding during the diarrhoeal episode;
- appropriate feeding during convalescence, with follow-up;
- effective communication of dietary instructions to the mother.

The first of these is considered in Unit 3; the remaining three topics are discussed below.

Feeding during diarrhoea

Specific feeding recommendations are determined by the child's age and pre-illness feeding pattern. These are summarized in Table 7.1 and discussed below.

Table 7.1 **Feeding of infants and children with acute diarrhoea**

Pre-illness feeding	Age in months		
	0–3	4–5	6 or more
Breast milk	Continue	Continue	Continue
Animal milk or formula[a]	Continue as usual	Continue as usual	Continue as usual
Soft or solid foods[a]	None	Continue if normally given	Continue, or start if not yet given

[a] These foods are not given during rehydration, but should be resumed immediately thereafter.

Breast milk

During diarrhoea, breast-feeding should not be reduced or stopped, but allowed as often and for as long as the infant desires it. Breast milk should be given in addition to ORS solution, a recommended home fluid, or other fluids given to replace stool losses.

Animal milk or formula

The infant should continue to receive the usual animal milk or formula. If dehydration develops, milk feeds should be stopped for 4–6 hours during rehydration, and then resumed. Special lactose-free or hydrolysed-protein formulas should not be used routinely; they are expensive and of no special value for most infants with acute diarrhoea. Occasionally, however, diarrhoea becomes worse when milk is given and signs of dehydration may appear. In such cases, the recommendations for the diagnosis and treatment of milk intolerance, given later in this unit (see opposite), should be followed.

Soft or solid foods

If the child is 4 months or older and already taking soft or solid foods these should be continued. Infants 6 months or older should be started on soft foods, if this has not already been done. If dehydration develops, these foods should be stopped for 4–6 hours during rehydration, and then resumed. At least half of the dietary energy should come from foods other than milk. Children should be given frequent small meals (e.g. six or more times per day) and they should be encouraged to eat. Guidelines for the selection of appropriate foods are given below.

- Use well-cooked local staple foods that can be easily digested, such as rice, corn, sorghum, potatoes, or noodles.

- Give the staple food in a soft, mashed form; for infants use a thick pap; if soups are given to prevent dehydration, other nutrient-rich foods must be given to ensure adequate caloric intake.

- Increase the energy content of the staple food by adding 5–10 ml of vegetable oil per 100 ml serving; red palm oil is especially good because it is also a rich source of carotene.

- Mix the staple food with well-cooked pulses and vegetables; if possible, include eggs, meat, or fish.

- Give fresh fruit juice, green coconut water, or mashed ripe banana to provide potassium.

- Avoid foods and drinks with a high concentration of sugar (e.g. sweetened commercial fruit drinks, soft drinks).

Milk intolerance

A few children with acute diarrhoea, especially young infants, show symptoms of intolerance of animal milk. This usually occurs when animal milk or formula is the only food given. Milk intolerance occurs more frequently among children with persistent diarrhoea (see Unit 6). It almost never occurs in children whose only milk is breast milk.

The clinical manifestations of milk intolerance are:

- a marked increase in stool volume and frequency when milk feeds are given, and a comparable decrease when they are stopped;
- worsening of the child's clinical condition; signs of dehydration may develop.

When milk intolerance is due to lactose malabsorption, the stool pH is low (less than 5.5; it turns litmus paper from blue to pink) and it contains a large amount of reducing substances (unabsorbed sugars). To test for reducing substances, add 8 drops of centrifuged fresh liquid stool to 5 ml of Benedict's solution and boil the mixture for 5 minutes; an orange-brown colour indicates that the stool contains more than 0.5% reducing substances. Clinitest tablets can also be used, but not most testing tapes, because they only detect glucose.

Be aware, however, that milk intolerance is often overdiagnosed. Stool volume and frequency may increase slightly when children with diarrhoea are fed aggressively; reducing substances may also appear in the stool and the faecal pH may become low. However, as long as the child is doing well clinically (i.e. is gaining weight, eating, alert, and active), these findings are not a cause for concern.

To manage milk intolerance:

- Continue breast-feeding.

- For infants under 4–6 months of age who take animal milk:
  - —replace cow's milk or formula with yoghurt or a similar fermented milk product, or dilute milk or formula with an equal volume of water (add 8 g of sugar to each 100 ml to maintain energy content); provide small feeds every 2–3 hours;
  - —if there is no improvement after 2 days, refer the infant to a centre where specialized treatment is possible. A lactose-free or milk-free diet may be required.

- For infants and children who normally take soft foods with animal milk:
  - —give only half the usual amount of animal milk or replace it with yoghurt or a similar fermented milk product;
  - —give sufficient amounts of well-cooked cereals, pulses and vegetables, with added vegetable oil, to ensure a normal caloric intake. Give these foods *mixed* with milk;
  - —if there is no improvement after 2 days, stop *all* animal milk products, replacing them with other energy-rich, protein-containing foods, such as a soya-based formula or finely minced chicken meat.

- Continue the treatment for milk intolerance for 2 days after diarrhoea has stopped, then reintroduce the usual milk or formula gradually over 2–3 days.

Feeding during convalescence, and follow-up

The child's usual diet should be reviewed and the mother advised on how she can improve its quality. In general, the foods recommended during diarrhoea should be continued after diarrhoea stops, and extra food should be given to support "catch up" growth. A practical approach is to give the child as much as he or she can eat and to provide an extra meal each day for 2 weeks. If the child is malnourished or is recovering from persistent diarrhoea, this should be continued for a longer period, until the malnutrition is corrected.

Ideally, the child should be seen regularly for follow-up so that his or her weight can be monitored, and encouragement and advice on feeding given to the mother. If possible, a *growth chart* should be used, especially if the child is malnourished, and follow-up continued until a normal rate of growth is established (see Annex 2). If these steps are not possible, the importance of giving extra food during convalescence and how to improve the quality of the child's usual diet should be explained to the mother; the best, and sometimes the only opportunity to do this is when the child is being treated for diarrhoea.

Vitamin A deficiency and diarrhoea

During diarrhoea, vitamin A absorption is reduced and greater amounts are used from body stores. In areas where vitamin A deficiency is a problem, diarrhoea can cause a rapid depletion of vitamin A stores, leading to acute vitamin A deficiency and symptoms or signs of xerophthalmia. Sometimes blindness develops rapidly. This is a particular problem when diarrhoea occurs during or shortly after measles, or in children who are already severely malnourished; it also occurs in children who have persistent diarrhoea or frequent episodes of diarrhoea.

Accordingly, children with diarrhoea who live in an area where vitamin A deficiency is a significant problem should be examined for symptoms and signs of vitamin A deficiency (see Unit 3). If night blindness is present or there are any signs of xerophthalmia, 200 000 units of vitamin A should be given by mouth; infants should receive 100 000 units. This dose should be repeated the next day and again after

2 weeks. Children who have severe malnutrition or have had measles within the past month should receive a single dose of vitamin A, as above (unless a dose has been given within the past month).

In areas where vitamin A deficiency is a problem, mothers should be encouraged to give their children foods rich in carotene, the precursor of vitamin A: these include yellow or orange vegetables and fruits (e.g. carrots, pumpkins, mangoes, yellow sweet potatoes, yellow bananas) and dark-green leafy vegetables.

Management of diarrhoea in children with severe malnutrition

Diarrhoea is a serious and often fatal event in children with severe malnutrition. Although the main objectives in treating such patients are the same as for better-nourished children, certain aspects of patient evaluation and management should be modified or given particular attention. These are described below. The diagnosis of severe malnutrition is described in Unit 3.

Assessment of hydration status

Assessment of hydration status in severely malnourished children is difficult, because a number of the signs normally used are unreliable. For example, children with marasmus have loose, lax skin and very little subcutaneous fat; their skin turgor appears poor, even when they are not dehydrated. On the other hand, skin turgor may appear normal in children with oedema (kwashiorkor), even when they are dehydrated. Likewise, sunken eyes are an unreliable sign in marasmic children; and the apathy of children with kwashiorkor and the irritable, fussy behaviour of those with marasmus make the interpretation of mental state difficult. Absence of tears is difficult to assess in all children with severe malnutrition because they do not readily cry. Signs that remain useful for detecting dehydration include: dry mouth and tongue, and eagerness to drink (for children with some dehydration); or very dry mouth and tongue, cool and moist extremities, and weak or absent radial pulse (for those with severe dehydration). In children with severe malnutrition it is often not possible to distinguish reliably between some dehydration and severe dehydration.

Rehydration therapy

The guidelines for rehydrating children with diarrhoea and severe malnutrition are as follows:

- Rehydration therapy should take place at a hospital, if possible; if the patient is seen at a health centre or clinic, he or she should be referred to hospital. The mother should be provided with ORS solution and shown how to give it to the child at a rate of 5 ml per kg of body weight per hour during the trip (see Fig. 6.1, page 82).

- All fluids should be given by mouth or nasogastric tube. Intravenous infusions should *not* be used because fluid overload occurs very easily, causing heart failure, and their use also increases the risk of septicaemia; either event is likely to be fatal. Oral rehydration is preferred for children who can drink; otherwise, a nasogastric tube should be used until the child is able to drink.

- Rehydration should be done slowly, over a period of 12–24 hours. The approximate amount of ORS solution to be given during this period is 70–100 ml per kg of body weight. The exact amount should be determined by the quantity the child will drink and by frequent, careful observation of the child for signs of overhydration (increasing oedema). The child should remain at the treatment centre until rehydration is completed.

- The standard ORS solution should be used. However, additional potassium should be given by mouth, since severely malnourished children are normally potassium-depleted, and this is made worse by diarrhoea. A convenient solution, containing 1 mmol of potassium per ml of solution, can be prepared by dissolving 7.5 g of potassium chloride in 100 ml of water; 4 ml of this solution per kg of body weight should be given each day for 2 weeks, in divided doses mixed with food.

- Feeding should be resumed as soon as possible. Fasting, even for brief periods, should be avoided. Breast-feeding should continue throughout rehydration and other food should be given as soon as it can be taken. Small amounts can usually be given within 2–3 hours after starting rehydration. The feeding guidelines given below should be followed.

Feeding

Children with severe malnutrition and diarrhoea must be fed very carefully; once rehydration is complete, nutritional rehabilitation should take place, preferably at a treatment centre with expertise in this area. Typically, children must spend 12–14 hours a day at the centre for feeding and supportive care, returning each night to their homes, where frequent feeding is continued. If the child must be admitted to hospital, the mother should stay, if possible, to assist with feeding and provide emotional support. For children with *kwashiorkor*, feeding should be resumed slowly, starting at 50–60 kcal per kg of body weight per day and reaching 110 kcal/kg per day after about 7 days; feeding usually has to be encouraged owing to the child's lack of interest in eating. For children with *marasmus*, feeding should be limited to 110 kcal/kg per day for the first week, but food can usually be given *ad libitum* thereafter. Semi-liquid or liquid foods must be given in numerous small feedings, e.g. every 2 hours, day and night. Initially, eating may be difficult because of stomatitis; in such instances, the child must be fed by nasogastric tube for several days.

A practical diet for initial feeding can be prepared from:

—skim milk powder 8 g;
—vegetable oil 6 g;
—sugar 5 g;
—water to make 100 ml.

This contains 100 kcal per 100 ml. If possible, the skim milk should be prepared first and fermented to make a yoghurt-like drink before the sugar and oil are added. This reduces the lactose content of the diet, so that it is better tolerated. The diet may also be prepared using fresh skim milk (briefly boiled) in place of skim milk powder and water. The oil is an important ingredient, as the diet would otherwise provide insufficient energy.

In addition, the following mineral and vitamin supplements should be given:

- iron — 60 mg of elemental iron per day;
- folic acid — 100 μg per day;
- vitamin A — 200 000 units once (100 000 units for infants) in areas where vitamin A deficiency is prevalent. If signs of xerophthalmia are present, the full treatment course described earlier (see page 102) should be given;
- vitamin B complex, vitamin C, and vitamin D — as daily multivitamin drops.

Further information on the nutritional management of children with severe malnutrition can be found in: *The treatment and management of severe protein–energy malnutrition,* Geneva, World Health Organization, 1981.

Associated illnesses

Children with severe malnutrition and diarrhoea frequently have other serious illnesses, especially infections. Most common are pneumonia, septicaemia, otitis media, pharyngitis, tonsillitis, and urinary or skin infections. Severe infection often causes hypothermia rather than fever. Patients should be examined carefully for evidence of infection and given appropriate antimicrobial therapy.

Talking with mothers about feeding during diarrhoea

Most societies have strong cultural beliefs about the feeding of infants and children during and after diarrhoea. Feeding recommendations must be nutritionally sound, but also compatible with the mother's beliefs and resources. In order to give effective dietary recommendations, the doctor must know:

- what foods are most commonly used for children at different ages and the nutritional value of these foods when prepared in the usual manner;
- what foods are commonly given or specifically prohibited during diarrhoea;
- what specific combinations can be recommended for nutrient-rich, low-bulk, soft, or semi-liquid diets, using foods that are available, acceptable, and affordable;
- how much food should be given to children with diarrhoea.

The doctor should ask the mother about the child's usual diet and about the food the child has received since diarrhoea began. The advice given should cover feeding both during diarrhoea and after diarrhoea stops; if possible, the recommendations for these two periods should be similar, with emphasis on a balanced, nutrient-rich diet that is appropriate for the child's age. If the mother does not have or cannot obtain the recommended foods, or is strongly opposed to giving certain items, the doctor should adjust the recommendations to fit her situation. If she does not know how to prepare certain foods, the doctor should ensure that she is given clear instructions and is able to follow them (see "Talking with mothers about home treatment", Unit 4).

Exercises

1. Which one of the following is the *most* important cause of weight loss during diarrhoea?

A. Reduced absorption of nutrients.
B. Increased metabolic demands.
C. Vomiting.
D. Anorexia.
E. Reduced intake of food.

2. Which of the following statements about feeding during diarrhoea are correct? (There may be more than one correct answer.)

   A. Feeding during diarrhoea does not appreciably increase stool volume.
   B. Continuing feeding during diarrhoea helps to hasten repair of the intestinal mucosa, thus restoring the production of disaccharidase enzymes.
   C. Food should be withheld when a child has anorexia.
   D. Special foods should be given during acute diarrhoea; the diet is not the same as that recommended when the child is well.
   E. Doctors should insist that mothers follow their advice about feeding, irrespective of the mothers' beliefs about what foods should or should not be given during diarrhoea.

3. Yunus, aged 9 months, is brought to you with watery, non-bloody diarrhoea, which he has had for 2 days. He has vomited twice. Physical examination shows evidence of some dehydration. You rehydrate him with ORS solution. His mother says that she stopped breast-feeding Yunus when she became pregnant 2 months ago. Since then, he has been taking cow's milk and eating rice with the rest of the family. When he started to have diarrhoea, she stopped his food.

   Which of the following points should be included in your advice to Yunus's mother? (There may be more than one correct answer.)

   A. Continue to give Yunus his normal milk feeds.
   B. Add 5–10 ml of vegetable oil to each serving of well-cooked rice.
   C. Add well-cooked pulses and vegetables to Yunus's diet; give him an egg, or some fish or meat when possible.
   D. Gradually resume Yunus's usual diet as the diarrhoea gets better.
   E. Give an extra meal each day for at least 2 weeks after diarrhoea stops.

4. Which of the following statements about feeding *after* acute diarrhoea are correct? (There may be more than one correct answer.)

   A. An extra meal should be given each day for at least 2 weeks.
   B. Milk should be withheld for several days, to prevent diarrhoea from returning.
   C. The foods given should be of the same type recommended for use during diarrhoea, i.e. nutrient-rich mixtures of a staple food, vegetable oil, pulses, vegetables and, if possible, meat, fish or egg. The usual milk should be given.
   D. Normal feeding should be resumed gradually, to prevent diarrhoea from returning.

5. Roberto, aged 9 months, has had frequent episodes of diarrhoea. He cries a lot and is restless during the examination. His skin pinch goes back slowly, he drinks eagerly, and his tongue is dry. His mother says that he has had diarrhoea frequently, "almost every month". He has been taking cow's milk from a feeding

bottle since he was 1 month old, and he started to take soft and semi-solid food at the age of 8 months. His mother says that he seems to be growing slowly, he does not need larger clothes as often as her previous children did, and he has been wearing the same protective charm bracelet on his wrist since he was 4 months old. Since the diarrhoea started his mother has given him some milk, but no solid food "because he was not hungry".

Roberto weighs 4.7 kg and has a "skin and bones" appearance. It is obvious that he is severely malnourished. What should be done for Roberto? (There may be more than one correct answer.)

A. He should be rehydrated orally with ORS solution at a rate of 70–100 ml/kg over 12–24 hours.
B. Food should be withheld until rehydration is completed.
C. If Roberto does not take the estimated volume of ORS solution, the remainder should be given intravenously as Ringer's lactate solution.
D. Roberto's treatment, including rehydration and nutritional management, should be given at a hospital or specialized treatment centre.
E. Roberto should be given supplemental potassium (a solution of potassium chloride added to his food) for 2 weeks.

6. *Part 1*: Kati is 7 months old. She is brought to you after 2 days with diarrhoea and has signs of severe dehydration. You initiate intravenous rehydration and then obtain further information from her mother. She says Kati was weaned to cow's milk 6 weeks earlier. Kati also eats well-cooked rice and vegetables and has continued to receive this diet during her illness. After rehydration you advise Kati's mother on home treatment, namely, feeding with cow's milk, rice, vegetables, and added oil. After 2 days, Kati's mother returns because Kati is still having frequent watery stools. The mother thinks these usually occur shortly after Kati takes milk. You think Kati may have milk intolerance. What *one* step would help *most* to confirm this diagnosis?

A. Stop all food for 2 days and see whether the diarrhoea improves.
B. Withhold milk for 12 hours (while continuing to give other foods) to see whether diarrhoea subsides, then give it again to see whether the diarrhoea promptly worsens.
C. Test the stool for pH and reducing substances.
D. Give a special soya-based milk and see whether the diarrhoea stops.
E. Give an antimicrobial and see whether the diarrhoea stops.

Part 2: If the diagnosis of milk intolerance is confirmed, what steps would be appropriate for its treatment? (There may be more than one correct answer.)

A. Give a special soya-based formula until the diarrhoea stops.
B. Give Kati only half of her usual amount of animal milk.
C. Provide at least half of Kati's food energy as cooked cereal and vegetables, with added vegetable oil. Mix Kati's milk with these foods.
D. Give yoghurt or another fermented milk product in place of milk.
E. Replace Kati's milk with fruit juice or tea.

UNIT 8

Prevention of diarrhoea

Introduction

Proper case management, consisting of oral rehydration therapy and feeding, can reduce the adverse effects of diarrhoea, which include dehydration, nutritional damage, and risk of death. Other measures are required, however, if the *incidence* of diarrhoeal episodes is to be substantially reduced; these include interventions that either reduce the spread of the microorganisms that cause diarrhoea or increase the child's resistance to infection with these agents. Prevention of diarrhoea, properly carried out, can be as important as case management, and may be the only way of avoiding deaths where treatment is not readily available.

A number of interventions have been proposed for preventing diarrhoea in young children, most of which involve measures related to infant feeding practices, personal hygiene, cleanliness of food, provision of safe water, safe disposal of faeces, and immunization. An analysis of the effectiveness, feasibility, and cost of each proposed intervention has shown that some are particularly effective and affordable, whereas others are impractical or ineffective, or require further evaluation. The review[1] concluded that efforts to prevent diarrhoea, and thus to reduce deaths not prevented by proper case management, should focus on a few interventions of proven efficacy. The seven practices identified as targets for promotion are:

- breast-feeding;
- improved weaning practices;
- use of plenty of water for hygiene and use of clean water for drinking;
- hand-washing;
- use of latrines;
- safe disposal of the stools of young children;
- measles immunization.

These topics are considered in detail in this unit.

Breast-feeding

Although breast milk is the best and safest food for young infants, the incidence of breast-feeding is declining in most developing countries. The reasons for this decline include the belief that bottle-feeding is "modern", the aggressive promotion of infant formulas, the need for mothers to work away from their children, the lack of facilities for breast-feeding at places of work, fear of not being able to breast-feed adequately, and a lack of medical and nursing support for mothers who want to breast-feed.

Nearly all women can breast-feed satisfactorily and breast-feeding has many benefits for both infant and mother (Fig. 8.1). Some major benefits are that breast-fed babies have fewer and less severe episodes of diarrhoea, and a lower risk of dying from diarrhoea than babies who are not breast-fed. For example, during the first 6 months of life, the risk of having severe diarrhoea that requires admission to hospital can be 30 times greater for infants who are not breast-fed than for those who are *exclusively* breast-fed (Fig. 8.2).

[1]Feachem, R.G. Preventing diarrhoea: what are the policy options? *Health policy and planning*, **1**: 109–117 (1986).

Fig. 8.1 **Breast-feeding has many advantages for both infant and mother**

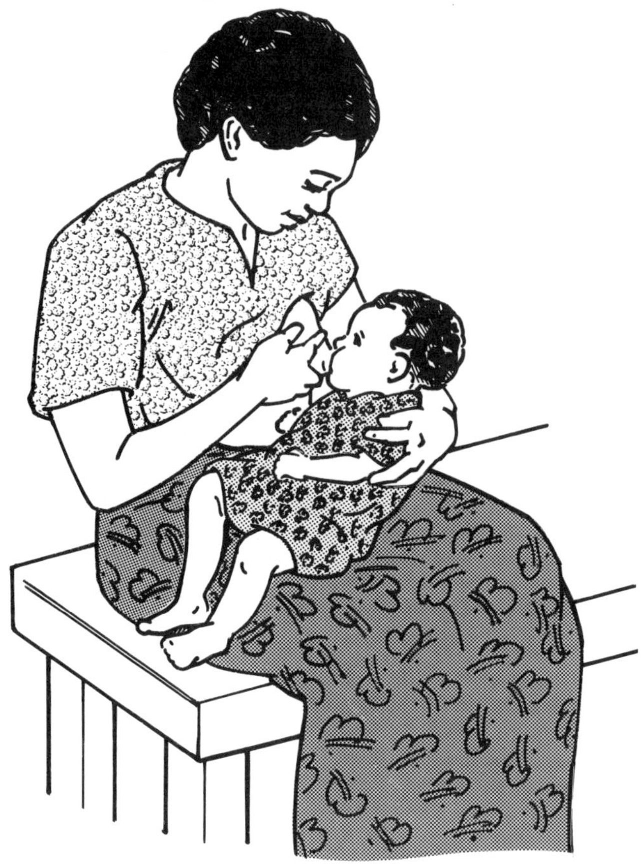

Important advantages of breast-feeding are:

- Exclusive breast-feeding during the first 4–6 months greatly reduces the risk of severe or fatal diarrhoea; the risk of other serious infections is also reduced.
- Breast-feeding is clean; it does not require the use of bottles, teats, water, and formula, which are easily contaminated with bacteria that may cause diarrhoea.
- Breast milk has immunological properties (especially antibodies) that protect the infant from infection, and especially from diarrhoea; these are not present in animal milk or formula.
- The composition of breast milk is ideal for the infant; formula or cow's milk may be made too dilute (which reduces its nutritional value) or too concentrated (so that it does not provide sufficient water) and may provide too much salt and sugar.
- Breast milk is a complete food; *it provides all the nutrients and water needed by a healthy infant during the first 4–6 months of life.* (However, low-birth-weight infants benefit from the provision of iron, if available.)
- Breast-feeding is cheap; there are none of the expenses associated with feeding breast-milk substitutes, e.g. the costs of fuel, utensils, and special formulas, and of the mother's time in formula preparation.

Fig. 8.2 **Relative risk of severe diarrhoea during the first 6 months of life**

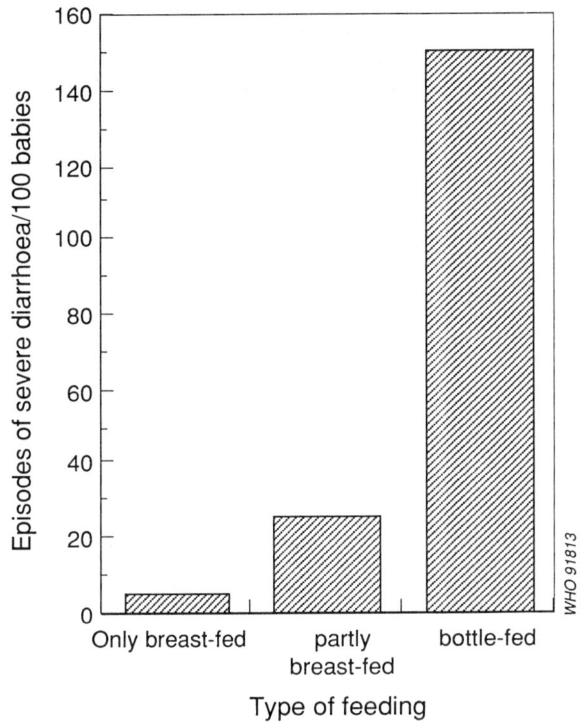

Source: Mahmood, D.A. et al. Infant feeding and risk of severe diarrhoea in Basrah city, Iraq: a case-control study. *Bulletin of the World Health Organization*, **67**: 701–706 (1989).

- Breast-feeding helps with birth spacing; mothers who breast-feed usually have a longer period of infertility after giving birth than mothers who do not breast-feed.
- Milk intolerance rarely occurs in infants who take only breast milk.
- Breast-feeding immediately after delivery encourages the "bonding " of the mother to her infant, which has important emotional benefits for both and helps to secure the child's place within the family.

If possible, infants should be *exclusively* breast-fed during the first 4–6 months of life. This means that a healthy baby who is growing normally should receive *only breast milk* and *no other fluids or foods such as water, tea, juices, or formula.*

Between 4 and 6 months of age, infants should start to receive cereals and other foods to meet their increased nutritional requirements, but breast-feeding should be continued at least until 2 years of age. Breast milk given after the age of 6 months is an important source of nutrients and it continues to help protect the child against episodes of severe diarrhoea.

Efforts to promote breast-feeding are especially important during pregnancy, at the time of birth (breast-feeding should begin as soon as possible after birth) and when problems are encountered after breast-feeding has been established. Most of these difficulties can be easily managed. Some ways of helping mothers to overcome problems related to breast-feeding are summarized in Table 8.1.

Table 8.1 **Common difficulties with breast-feeding**

If the mother:	Then the health worker should:
Says she does not have enough breast milk	Determine whether the baby is gaining weight normally: • If the baby's weight gain is normal, try to find out why the mother is anxious. Reassure her that her baby is growing normally and that she is producing enough milk. • If the baby's weight gain is less than normal, suggest that she tries to increase the supply of milk by breast-feeding as often and as long as the baby wants, at least 6–8 times a day. If the baby still does not gain weight, supplement the breast milk with formula, offering it *after* the breast-feed. If the infant is at least 4 months old, supplement the milk with cereal, well-cooked vegetables, and other weaning foods (see Unit 7).
Has a sore or cracked nipple	Show her how to continue to breast-feed without injuring the nipple. Tell her to: • Make sure that when the baby feeds, the nipple *and the areola* are in the baby's mouth. The gums should close on the areola, *not* on the nipple. • Feed the baby frequently from the breast with the sore nipple. • Change the position of the baby so the baby's mouth does not always hold the breast in the same way. • Let the nipple dry in the air after breast-feeding or expressing milk. If she cannot breast-feed because of pain, show her how to express her milk manually and feed it to her baby.
Has an engorged breast (the breast is too full of milk)	Show her how to express milk manually. Tell her to breast-feed frequently.
Has an infected breast (signs of infection include a swollen, painful, and reddened breast with tender lymph nodes under the arm)	Give her an appropriate antimicrobial (e.g. penicillin). Tell her to continue breast-feeding and explain that milk from the infected breast is still safe for her baby. Start feedings on the unaffected breast, then move the infant to the affected breast after milk let-down has occurred. Severe pain may require the expression of some milk by hand.

What mothers should do

- Start breast-feeding as soon as possible after delivery.
- Breast-feed the baby exclusively, if possible, for the first 4–6 months, and continue breast-feeding for at least 2 years.
- Breast-feed on demand; more frequent sucking causes the milk supply to increase.
- If it is not possible to take the baby to work, breast-feed before leaving home, on returning home, at night, and at any other time when the mother is with the baby.
- Express milk manually to avoid engorgement of the breasts during periods of separation from the baby.

- Continue breast-feeding during and after any illness of the baby, especially diarrhoea.

What doctors should do

- Encourage hospital policies and routine procedures after delivery that promote the breast-feeding of neonates. For example, allow mothers to start breast-feeding immediately after delivery; keep all healthy babies close to their mothers in the same room (termed "rooming-in"); do not allow any food or fluids except breast milk to be given to newborns; do not distribute (or allow sales representatives or nurses to distribute) samples of milk formula or feeding bottles to the mothers.

Improved weaning practices

Weaning is the process by which an infant gradually becomes accustomed to an adult diet. During weaning, supplementary foods other than milk are introduced in order to meet the child's increased nutritional demands. However, breast milk remains an important part of the diet.

Weaning is a hazardous period for many infants. This is because the child may not receive food of adequate nutritional value and the food and drinks provided may be contaminated with pathogenic microorganisms, including those that cause diarrhoea. The danger is that the child will become malnourished due to an inadequate diet and repeated episodes of diarrhoea, or will succumb to dehydration caused by an acute episode of diarrhoea. Unfortunately, these processes are interrelated: malnutrition increases the child's susceptibility to infection so that the child experiences more prolonged and more severe episodes of diarrhoea, and diarrhoea accelerates the development of malnutrition (see Fig. 7.2, page 96).

Some specific problems associated with weaning that can lead to malnutrition or diarrhoea are:

- delaying the start of weaning beyond 4–6 months of age;
- weaning too abruptly;
- giving too few meals per day;
- giving supplementary foods with a low content of protein and energy;
- preparing and storing weaning foods in a way that permits bacterial contamination and growth;
- giving milk or other drinks prepared with contaminated water or in a contaminated feeding bottle.

What mothers should do

When to begin weaning

Weaning should begin when the child is 4–6 months old. While continuing to breast-feed, the mother should give a little well-cooked soft or mashed food, such as cereal and vegetables, twice each day. When the child is 6 months of age, the variety of foods should be increased and meals should be given *at least four times per day*, in addition to breast-feeding. After 1 year of age, the child should eat all types of food; vegetables, cereals, and meat should continue to be well cooked, and mashed or ground. Food should be given at least four times a day. If possible, breast-feeding should be continued.

What foods to give

Cereals and starchy roots are the most widely used weaning foods, but these are relatively low in energy. They should be given as a thick pap or porridge, using a spoon, and not as a dilute drink. The energy content should be increased by mixing one or two teaspoonfuls of vegetable oil into each serving. The objective is to achieve an energy intake of about 110 kcal/kg per day. Between the age of 6 months and 1 year, pulses, fruit, green vegetables, eggs, meat, fish, and milk products should be added to the diet.

In areas where vitamin A deficiency is a problem, the diet should include orange or yellow vegetables and fruits (see page 103), and dark-green leafy vegetables. Weaning foods are considered in greater detail in Unit 7.

Preparing and giving weaning foods

Mothers should be taught ways of preparing, giving, and storing weaning foods that minimize the risk of bacterial contamination. These include:

- Carefully washing the hands before preparing weaning foods and before feeding the baby.
- Preparing the food in a clean place.
- Cooking or boiling the food well.
- If possible, preparing the food immediately before it will be eaten.
- Covering food that is being kept. Keeping food in a cool place; refrigerating it if possible.
- If cooked food was prepared more than 2 hours before it is used, reheating it until it is thoroughly hot (and then allowing it to cool) before giving it to the baby.
- Feeding the baby with a clean spoon, from a cup, or with a special feeding spoon (Fig. 8.3). Feeding bottles should *never* be used.
- Washing uncooked food in clean water before feeding it to the baby; an exception is fruit that is peeled before it is eaten, such as a banana.

What doctors should do

- Make the assessment of weaning diets and weaning education a routine element of well-baby programmes. This should be coordinated with the use of growth charts to

Fig. 8.3 **How to feed liquids to an infant**

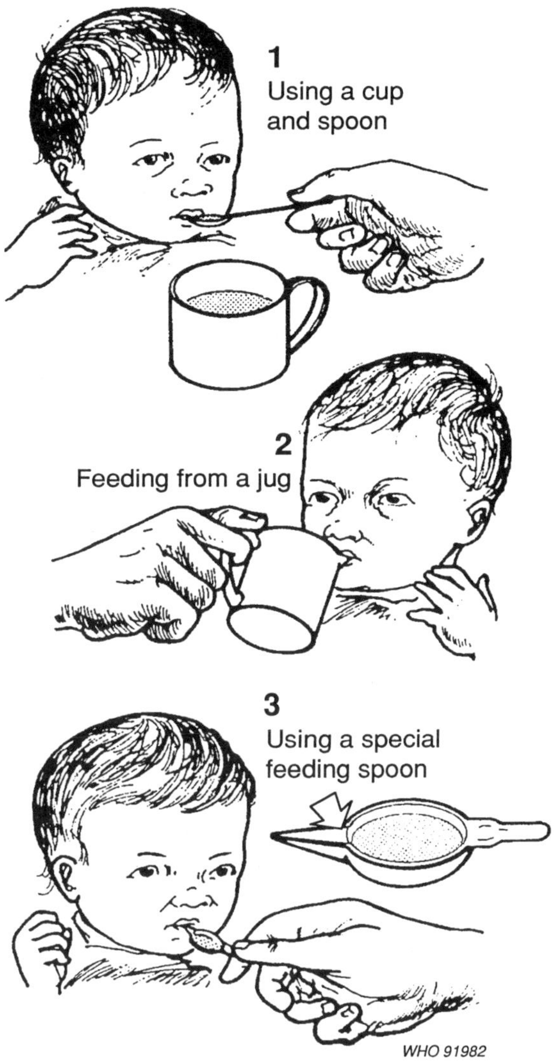

identify children with growth faltering, for whom improved feeding is especially important.

- Evaluate the nutritional status of children with diarrhoea, by measuring mid-upper arm circumference, weight-for-age, or weight-for-height:
  - —refer all children with severe malnutrition to a treatment centre where nutritional rehabilitation is possible;
  - —for moderately malnourished children, ask about the child's weaning diet and feeding practices. Advise the mother on ways of increasing the child's intake of safely prepared, nutrient-rich foods. If possible, follow up the child after the diarrhoea has stopped until the weight or rate of growth has become normal;
  - —otherwise, provide advice on correct feeding during and after the episode of diarrhoea (giving one extra meal each day for at least 2 weeks after the diarrhoea has stopped).

Proper use of water for hygiene and drinking

Most infectious agents that cause diarrhoea are transmitted by the faecal–oral route. This includes transmission by contaminated drinking-water or contaminated food, and from person to person. A plentiful supply of water helps to encourage hygienic practices, such as hand-washing, cleaning of eating utensils, and cleaning of latrines; these practices can interrupt the spread of infectious agents that cause diarrhoea. To facilitate good hygiene, it is more important that the water supply be abundant than clean, although both qualities are desirable. Clean water is essential, however, for drinking and for preparing food.

Families that have ready access to a generous supply of water, and to clean water for drinking and preparing food, have diarrhoea less frequently than families whose access to water is difficult or whose drinking-water is heavily contaminated. Improved water supplies can result from government-sponsored programmes, in which families and communities may play an important role, or from other community or family efforts, such as collecting and storing rainwater.

What families should do

- Use the most readily available water for personal and domestic hygiene. If this water is likely to be contaminated, store it separately from water used for drinking or preparing food.

- Collect drinking-water from the cleanest available source.

- Protect water sources by keeping animals away, by locating latrines more than 10 metres away and downhill, and by digging drainage ditches to divert stormwater.

- Collect and store drinking-water in clean containers. Keep the storage container covered and do not allow children or animals to drink from it. Do not allow anyone to put his or her hand into the storage container. Take out water only with a long-handled dipper that is kept especially for that purpose. Empty and rinse out the container every day.

- Boil water that will be used to make food or drinks for young children. Boil other drinking-water if sufficient fuel is available. Water needs to boil for only a few seconds; vigorous boiling is unnecessary and wastes fuel.

Hand-washing

Parents can help to protect young children against diarrhoea by adopting certain hygienic practices. One very important practice is hand-washing (Fig. 8.4). Hand-washing is especially effective for preventing the spread of *Shigella,* which is the most important cause of dysentery. For example, a study in Bangladesh[1] has shown that hand-washing with soap and water reduced the incidence of secondary cases of

[1] Khan, M.U. Interruption of shigellosis by hand-washing. *Transactions of the Royal Society of Tropical Medicine and Hygiene,* **76**: 164–168 (1982).

Fig. 8.4 **Hands should be washed carefully after defecation, before handling food and before eating**

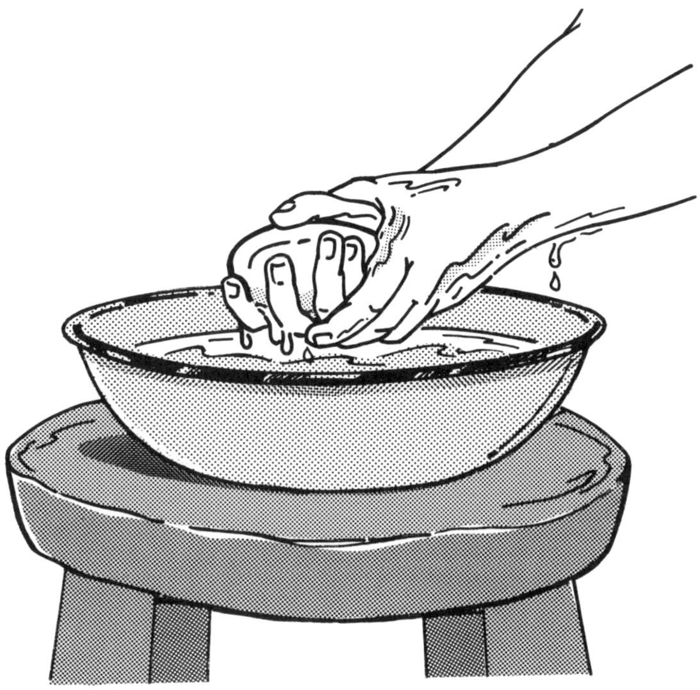

shigellosis by a factor of seven (from 14% to 2%) in households where a case of shigellosis had been detected.

Good hand-washing requires the use of soap (or a local substitute), plenty of water, and careful cleaning of all parts of the hands. If water is scarce, it can be used more than once to wash hands. It can then be used to wash the floor, to clean the latrine, or to irrigate the vegetable garden.

What families should do

- Create a place within the home for hand-washing. This should have a wash basin, a container for water, and soap (or a local substitute).
- All members should wash their hands well:

  —after cleaning a child who has defecated, or after disposing of a child's stool;
  —after defecating;
  —before preparing food;
  —before eating;
  —before feeding a child.

- An adult or older sibling should wash the hands of young children.

Use of latrines

Human faeces should be disposed of in a way that prevents them from coming into contact with hands or contaminating a water source. This is best achieved through regular use of a well-maintained latrine. The proper use of latrines can reduce the risk of diarrhoea to almost the same extent as improved water supplies, but the greatest benefit occurs when improvements in sanitation and water supply are combined and education is given on hygienic practices.

Every family should have and use a clean and well-maintained latrine. Families that do not have a latrine should be encouraged to build one, following a design recommended by the relevant government agency. If there is no latrine or pit, families should defecate as hygienically as possible, away from the path, and at least 10 metres away from any home or source of water. Consideration should be shown by not defecating in areas uphill or upstream from other people. If possible, faeces should be covered with dirt.

What families should do

- Have a clean, functioning latrine that is used by all members of the family old enough to do so. Keep the latrine clean by regularly washing down fouled surfaces.

- If there is no latrine:

  —defecate away from the house, and from areas where children play, and at least 10 metres from the water supply;
  —cover the faeces with earth;
  —do not allow children to visit the defecation area alone; keep children's hands off the ground near the defecation area.

Safe disposal of the stools of young children

In many communities the stools of infants and young children are considered harmless. However, young children are frequently infected with enteric pathogens and their stools are actually an important source of infection for others. This is true both for children with diarrhoea and for those with asymptomatic infections. Therefore, hygienic disposal of the faeces of *all* young children is an important aspect of diarrhoea prevention. Education is needed to warn families of the dangerous nature of young children's stools and to stress the importance of disposing of them properly.

What families should do

- Quickly collect the stool of a young child or baby, wrap it in a large leaf or newspaper, and put it in the latrine, or bury it.

- Help older children to defecate into a potty. Empty the stool immediately into a latrine and wash out the potty. Alternatively, have the child defecate onto a disposable surface, such as newspaper or a large leaf. Wrap up the stool and dispose of it in a latrine, or bury it.

- Promptly clean a child who has defecated. Then wash their own and the child's hands with soap and water.

Measles immunization

Children who have measles, or have had the disease in the previous 4 weeks, have a substantially increased risk of developing severe or fatal diarrhoea or dysentery (there is some evidence that the increased risk lasts up to 6 months after the measles episode). Because of the strong relationship between measles and serious diarrhoea, and the effectiveness of measles vaccine, immunization against measles is a very cost-effective measure for reducing the morbidity and mortality associated with diarrhoea. Measles vaccine given at the recommended age can prevent up to 25% of diarrhoea-associated deaths in children under 5 years of age.

What families should do

- Have children immunized against measles at the recommended age.

What doctors should do

- Include screening and referral for immunization, including measles immunization, as a routine practice in well-baby clinics.

- Ask mothers always to bring the child's immunization card when they come to the clinic for any reason. Check the immunization status of every patient and make sure that those who need it are immunized during the visit, unless there is a valid reason against it. Diarrhoea is *not* a reason to postpone immunization.

Talking with mothers about preventing diarrhoea

Most activities that help to prevent diarrhoea must take place in the home. However, mothers and other family members cannot practise diarrhoea prevention until they have learned what this involves and understand how best to carry out each preventive activity. Information on the prevention of diarrhoea can be provided in a variety of ways, e.g. at community meetings, through schools, during home visits and visits to a health centre. The latter may be especially effective when the visit involves a child with diarrhoea; at this time the mother is particularly aware of the problem of diarrhoea and is more likely to be interested in knowing what steps she can take to prevent future episodes. Care should be taken, however, not to overwhelm the mother with information, as she will also be given instructions concerning home treatment of her child. If possible, messages on prevention should focus on the interventions that are considered most desirable for the particular child; this is especially important for preventive measures that concern feeding, which will depend upon the child's age and feeding status.

Discussions with mothers about preventing diarrhoea should follow the same principles as those concerning home treatment of diarrhoea (Unit 4). They should be supportive and understanding, not critical. Remember that the goal is to help the mother to understand that she plays a very important role in assuring her child's health.

How doctors can help to prevent diarrhoea

Most of the interventions described in this unit involve education — of mothers in particular, but also of other family members. The objective is to achieve a change in behaviour that diminishes the risk of diarrhoea, usually by reducing the transmission of infectious agents. In many situations this effort will be organized and led by doctors, and much of the educational activity will occur at health facilities. Specific ways in which doctors can help to organize or strengthen such educational efforts include:

- *Ensuring appropriate in-service training of the health facility staff.* Most teaching of mothers about preventive measures, such as breast-feeding, weaning practices, hand-washing, and stool disposal, is carried out by health facility staff. Doctors should organize regular, in-service training of the staff to ensure that they understand the key messages mothers should receive and the most effective ways of conveying them. Staff should also be taught to practise appropriate preventive measures during their work, e.g. washing their hands with soap and water after examining a patient with diarrhoea.

- *Displaying promotional material on how to prevent diarrhoea.* Educational posters should be displayed in areas of the health facility where they can be used to teach mothers how to prevent diarrhoea. They should cover all the preventive measures considered in this unit.

- *Being a good role model.* Doctors should encourage in their own homes measures that prevent diarrhoea and protect the health of their children, such as exclusive breast-feeding for the first 4–6 months of life and continued breast-feeding for at least the first 2 years. They should ensure that the health facility and its staff are good role models for the community. For example, water should be stored and handled safely, facilities for hand-washing should be available and carefully maintained, and latrines should be well constructed and regularly cleaned.

- *Taking part in community-oriented activities to promote health.* Giving talks or taking part in community meetings is an effective way of promoting certain preventive measures, such as appropriate weaning practices, immunization against measles and other diseases, improvements in water supply and use, and construction and use of latrines.

- *Coordinating efforts for disease prevention with those of relevant government programmes.* Doctors should learn about and use the resources of government programmes concerned with disease prevention. This applies broadly to the areas of immunization, infant feeding practices, hygiene, sanitation, and water supply. These programmes are often valuable sources of teaching materials, such as wall posters or pamphlets for mothers, and may also provide guidelines for local practices, e.g. on the most appropriate weaning foods or designs for latrines.

Exercises

1. Which of the following measures are cost-effective with regard to the prevention of diarrhoea in young children? (There may be more than one correct answer.)

A. Control of flies.
B. Hand-washing after defecation, before preparing food, and before eating.
C. Exclusive breast-feeding for the first 4–6 months of life; continued breast-feeding for at least 2 years.
D. Immunizing against measles at the recommended age.

2. Which of the following statements concerning breast-feeding are correct? (There may be more than one correct answer.)

   A. The protection of breast-fed infants against diarrhoea is not affected when other foods or drinks are given.
   B. Breast-fed infants below 4 months of age do not need other foods, but should be given water or other drinks, especially if they live in a hot, dry climate.
   C. Infants who are exclusively breast-fed have a greatly reduced risk of developing severe diarrhoea compared with infants taking animal milk or formula from a bottle.
   D. Milk intolerance occurs with equal frequency in breast-fed and bottle-fed infants.

3. Many episodes of diarrhoea occur during the period of weaning, when malnutrition is also most prevalent. Which of the following factors help to cause diarrhoea and malnutrition during the weaning period? (There may be more than one correct answer.)

   A. Storing cooked weaning foods at room temperature for several hours; then giving them to the child without reheating them thoroughly.
   B. Giving weaning foods that have a low content of energy and protein.
   C. Not washing the hands before preparing the child's food.
   D. Giving milk or other drinks in a feeding bottle.
   E. Giving three meals a day to a 1-year-old child.

4. Which of the following statements concerning behaviour that is related to the prevention of diarrhoea are correct? (There may be more than one correct answer.)

   A. Stools of infants are less likely to cause disease than those of adults.
   B. Where water is scarce, it may be used more than once for washing hands.
   C. At 5 or 6 years of age, children need not use a latrine.
   D. After cleaning a baby who has defecated, it is important for a mother to wash her hands.
   E. It is important that the cleanest water available be used for *all* household purposes, such as bathing and washing clothes.

5. Hand-washing at appropriate times can help to prevent diarrhoea. Which of the following are important times for hand-washing? (There may be more than one correct answer.)

   A. Before eating.
   B. Before breast-feeding an infant.
   C. After defecating.
   D. After disposing of an infant's stool.
   E. Before drinking water.

ANNEX 1

Diarrhoea case record form

Registration No.__________ Admission Date______________ Hour__________
Discharge Date______________ Hour__________

Patient's Name:____________________________________ Age: _______Years _______Months

Address:____________________________________ Sex: ______

CHECK FOR SIGNS OF DEHYDRATION (Circle each sign that is present)

	PLAN A	PLAN B	PLAN C
1. LOOK AT: CONDITION	Well, alert	***Restless, irritable***	***Lethargic or unconscious; floppy***
EYES	Normal	Sunken	Very sunken and dry
TEARS	Present	Absent	Absent
MOUTH and TONGUE	Moist	Dry	Very dry
THIRST	Drinks normally, not thirsty	***Thirsty, drinks eagerly***	***Drinks poorly or not able to drink***
2. FEEL: SKIN PINCH	Goes back quickly	***Goes back slowly***	***Goes back very slowly***
3. DECIDE:	The patient has NO SIGNS OF DEHYDRATION	If the patient has two or more signs, including at least one ***sign***, there is SOME DEHYDRATION	If the patient has two or more signs, including at least one ***sign***, there is SEVERE DEHYDRATION

Treatment Plan Selected (circle one) A B C

If Plan B or C selected, weight of child________kg

CHECK FOR OTHER PROBLEMS

Duration of diarrhoea:___________days

Fever during last 5 days?__________Yes_____No

Blood seen in stool?_____Yes_____No

Current temperature:____________________

Signs of severe malnutrition?______Yes_____No

SPECIFY DETAILS OF TREATMENT

If Plan A, ask about the child's diet and advise the mother about home treatment (see page 3).

If Plan B, amount of ORS to give in first 4 hours: ____________________ml

If Plan C, amount of IV fluid to be given: __________in first _________minutes
__________in next_________hours

If IV therapy not possible (tick one):

_____ give ORS by nasogastric tube: _____ ml per hour

_____ give ORS by mouth to patient who can drink: _____ ml per hour

_____ refer patient to ________________________________

Medicines to give (name, dose and frequency):

1. ____

2. ____

Food to be given during treatment (including breast milk): ____

MONITOR PROGRESS OF PATIENT

Treatment of dehydration:

Type(s) of fluid given (IV or ORS)	Amount taken by patient	Time period when volumes were taken

Treatment for other problems:

Medicine given	Amount	Time given

Reassessment of hydration status:

Time	Signs of dehydration	Degree of dehydration and treatment plan needed

Food given during treatment (including breast milk):

Comments (Note any difficulties and how managed):

BEFORE DISCHARGE, ASK MOTHER ABOUT

Child's usual diet

Liquids

_____breast milk
_____animal milk
_____formula or powdered milk
_____other:_________________

Solid food

Foods taken daily__________________

____

Shares family food? _____Yes _____No
Number of meals each day __________

Diet since onset of diarrhoea

What types of fluid have been given at home since onset?
____
____

Has milk or formula been made with more water than usual? _____Yes _____No

Has the amount of fluid given been:

_______more than usual
_______the usual amount
_______less than usual
_______none given

Has the amount of food given been:

_______more than usual
_______the usual amount
_______less than usual
_______none given

Immunizations

Are immunizations up-to-date? _____Yes _____No
If NO, which vaccines are needed? ____

THEN ADVISE MOTHER ABOUT HOME TREATMENT

Was the mother taught how to make ORS solution? _____ Yes _____No

Number of ORS packets given: _____ Packet size: _____ml

Fluids to give:

Foods to give:

Other advice:

Discussed with mother the signs that mean the child should return? _____Yes _____No

IMMUNIZATIONS: Needed vaccines given or child referred for immunization? _____Yes _____No

Signature: ____

ANNEX 2
Growth chart

An example of a growth chart that can be used for plotting the changes in body weight of an infant or young child is shown opposite. As maintenance of good nutrition is important in the prevention of diarrhoea, an episode of diarrhoea is an excellent time to start using a growth chart, if one is not already being used.

The value of a growth chart is not to determine the nutritional status of a child at a particular time. Rather, its principal use is to monitor *growth over time* by measuring changes in weight (an example of a child's growth curve is shown on the chart opposite). The infant or young child should be weighed at regular intervals and the weight entered on the chart in the vertical column corresponding to the child's age. If the direction of the line joining successive weights is upwards and parallel to the solid lines (arrows A and C on the chart), the child is growing satisfactorily. A horizontal or downwards direction of the line (arrow B) is a sign of inadequate nutrition and/or illness. These patterns are especially helpful in the first year of life; in older children slight fluctuations in growth normally occur without signalling danger.

The curved lines that run across the chart show the *shape* of normal growth curves. The growth curves of most healthy children will lie between these lines or above the upper line. If a child's weight is much below the lower reference line there is some reason for concern. However, even in this case it is the direction of the child's growth curve that is most important.

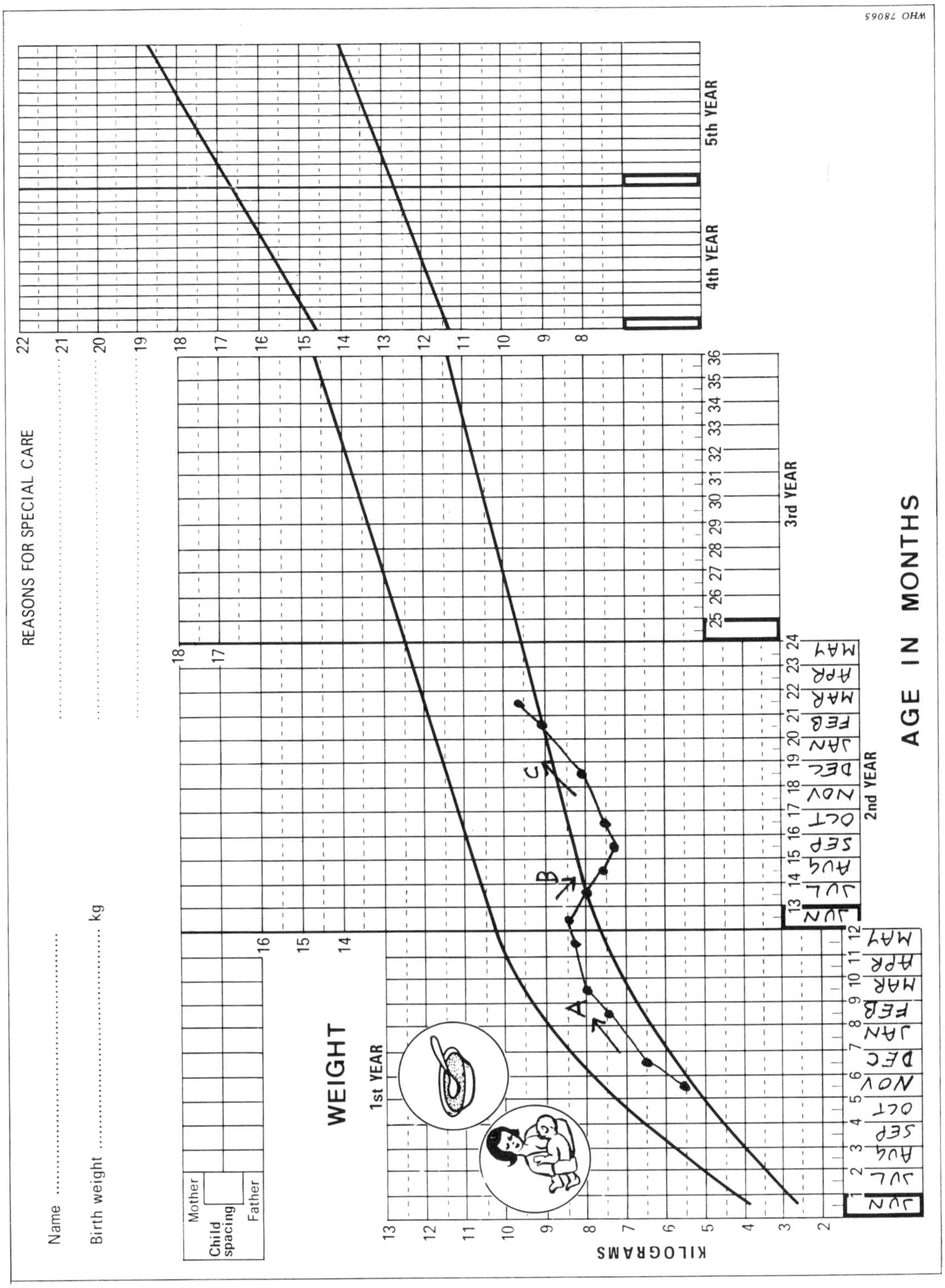
WHO 78065
Name
Birth weight kg
REASONS FOR SPECIAL CARE
Mother
Child spacing
Father
WEIGHT
KILOGRAMS
1st YEAR
2nd YEAR
3rd YEAR
4th YEAR
5th YEAR
AGE IN MONTHS
JUN JUL AUG SEP OCT NOV DEC JAN FEB MAR APR MAY
A
B
C

ANNEX 3

How to determine whether a child is malnourished

The upper arm has a bone, muscles and fat. When babies are about 1 year old, they have quite a lot of fat under the skin of their arms. When they are 5 years old, there is much less fat and more muscle. The distance around the upper arm remains almost the same between the ages of 1 and 5 years. If a child is malnourished, this distance is reduced, and the arm becomes thin. This is due to a reduction in muscle and fat. By placing a special measuring strip around the upper arm one can find out whether a child between the ages of 1 and 5 years is malnourished or not.

This measuring strip is called a tricoloured arm strip and looks like this:

A tricoloured arm strip

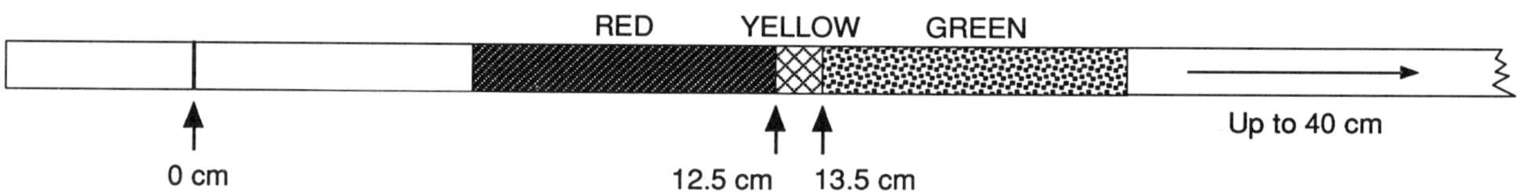

WHO 91978

You can make one from a strip of material that *does not stretch*, being careful that the markings are accurate.

To use this strip:

Put the strip around the mid upper arm of the child and see which colour is touched by the 0 cm mark on the strip.

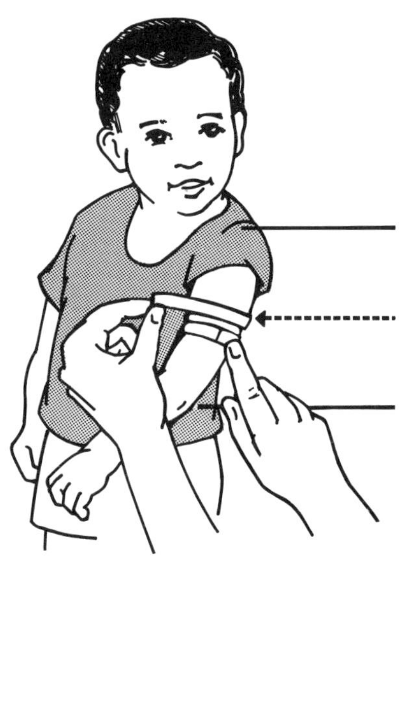

—If the green part is touched, the child is *well nourished.*
—If the yellow part is touched, the child is *moderately malnourished.*
—If the red part is touched, the child is *severely malnourished.*

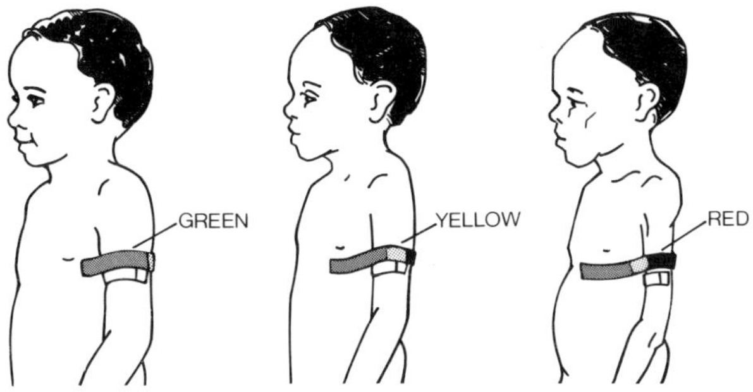

This method of measuring the arm is useful because the health worker can identify malnutrition in a child without using a scale or knowing the child's age. However, since it only shows large changes in a child's nutrition, it is not suitable for determining whether the child is improving or becoming worse.

ANNEX 4

Intravenous rehydration

Intravenous rehydration must only be performed using needles, administration sets, and IV fluids that are sterile. Administration sets should *never* be reused. Needles should be reused *only* if carefully cleaned and resterilized. Care must be taken to avoid contact with the patient's blood while starting an IV infusion.

A. Peripheral vein infusion

1. Lay the child in a comfortable position. Have an assistant hold the child.

2. Select a vein on the arm or leg that is easy to see; this is usually on the back of the hand or in the antecubital fossa.

3. Use a tourniquet to make the veins enlarge and select the largest vein.

4. Clean the skin with alcohol or soap and water.

5. Stretch the skin over the vein and gently insert the needle into the vein.

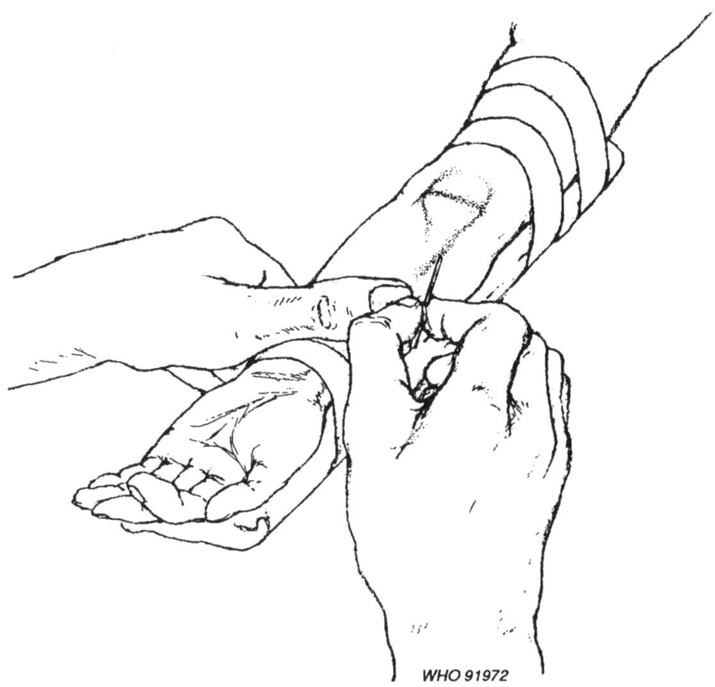

6. If the needle is in the vein, blood should fill the needle's opening. If it does not, gently reposition the needle.

7. Release the tourniquet and attach the IV tubing to the needle, having first run fluid from the IV bottle through the tubing to remove the air.

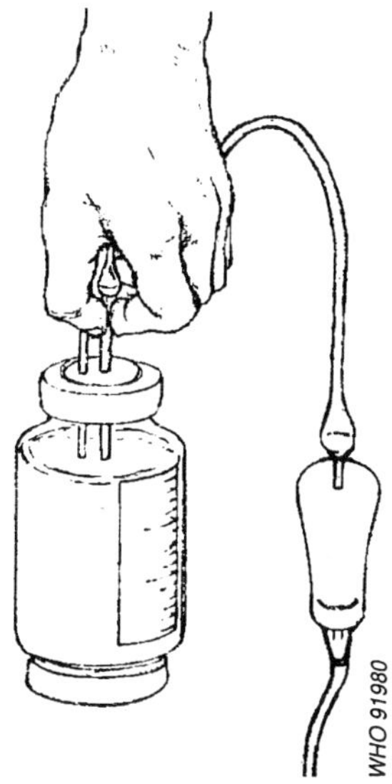

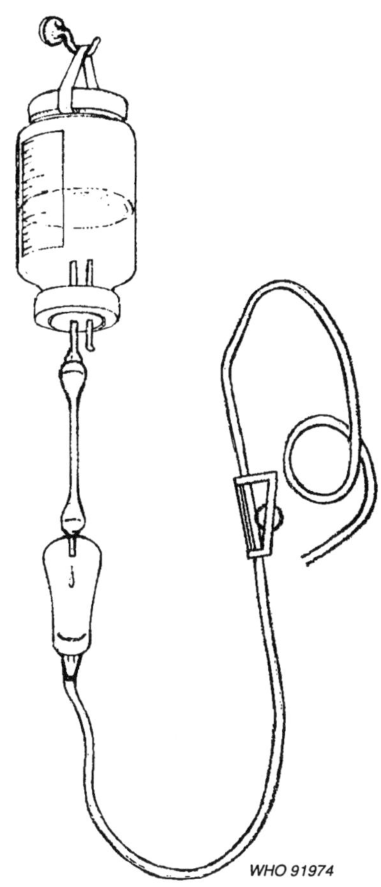

8. Slowly run 0.5–1 ml of fluid into the vein. If swelling occurs around the needle, remove it and start again further up the vein.

9. Fasten the needle and tubing firmly to the skin with adhesive tape. Use an arm board to keep the joint nearest the needle from moving.

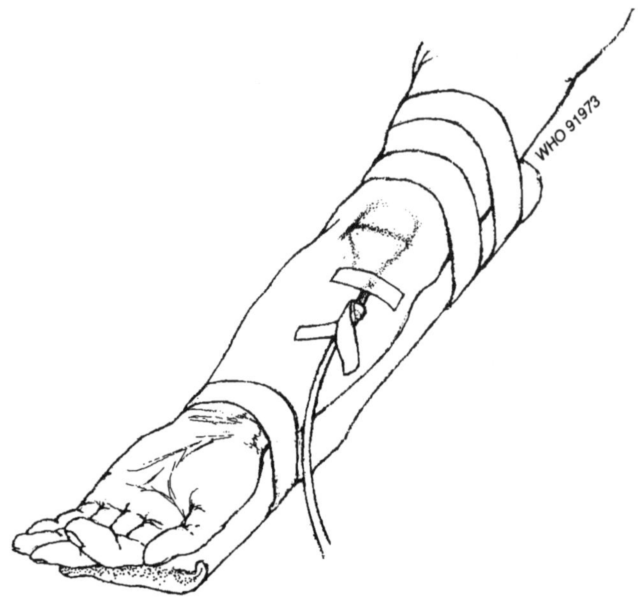

10. Regulate the flow of fluid and check again that there is no swelling around the needle.

11. Gently restrain the child's arms or legs so that the needle will not be dislodged by movement.

B. Scalp vein infusion

1. Wrap the child in a sheet or blanket, but not so tightly that breathing is restricted. Lay the child down and have an assistant hold the child.

2. Select a vein (usually behind the ear) and shave the scalp over the vein. Clean the shaved area with alcohol or soap and water.

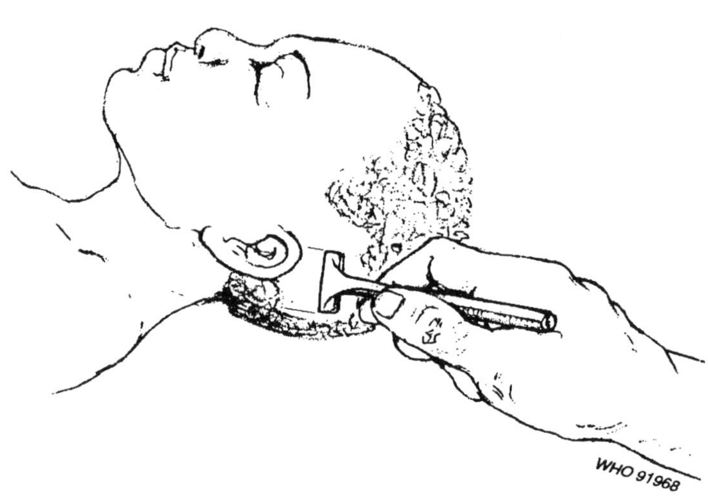

3. Stretch the skin over the vein and gently insert the scalp vein needle (or butterfly needle) into the vein. Placing a finger on the vein in front of where the needle will be inserted causes the vein to fill with blood and to be easier to enter.

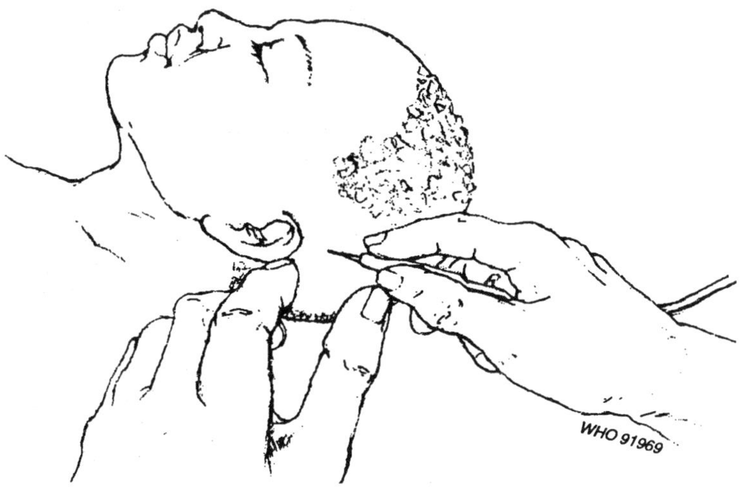

4. If the needle is in the vein, light pressure on the vein will cause the needle opening to fill with blood. If it does not, pull the needle back a bit.

5. When blood appears in the needle opening, connect the IV tubing to the needle, having first run fluid from the IV bottle through the tubing to remove the air.

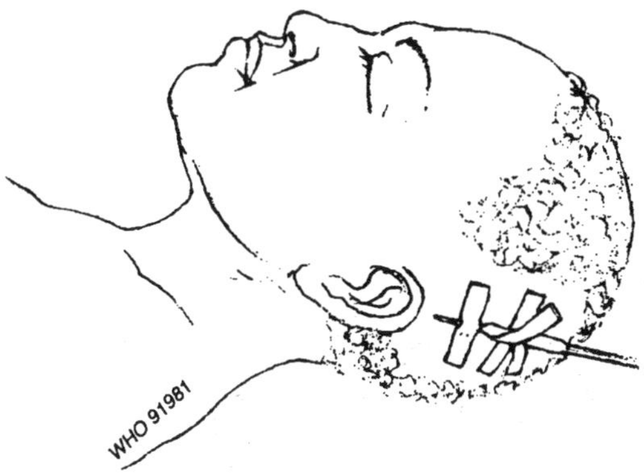

6. Slowly run 0.5–1 ml of fluid into the vein. If swelling occurs, remove the needle and start again with another vein.

7. Fasten the needle firmly in place with adhesive tape. If necessary, place a gauze pad under the needle hub to support it in a position that allows fluid to flow freely into the vein.

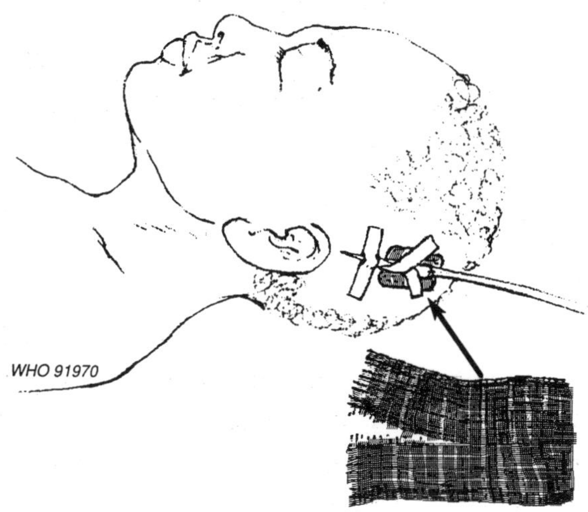

8. Regulate the flow of fluid and check again that there is no swelling around the needle.

9. Fasten the tubing to the child's head, leaving a loop as shown.

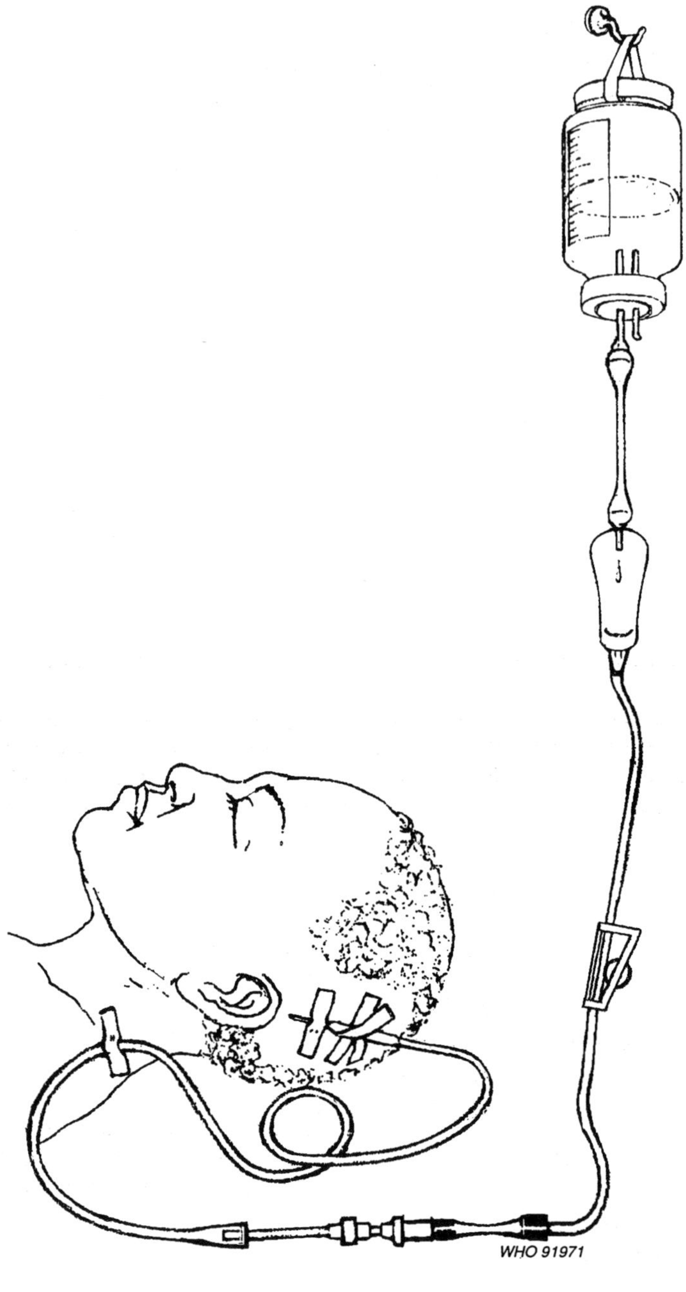

C. Femoral vein infusion

The femoral vein can be used as a temporary site for IV infusion in patients with severe hypovolaemia when no vein can be found in the arms, legs or scalp. After a rapid IV infusion to correct shock, the needle should be removed from the femoral vein and placed in a peripheral vein. The technique for inserting a needle in the femoral vein is shown opposite.

Technique for inserting an intravenous infusion needle into the femoral vein

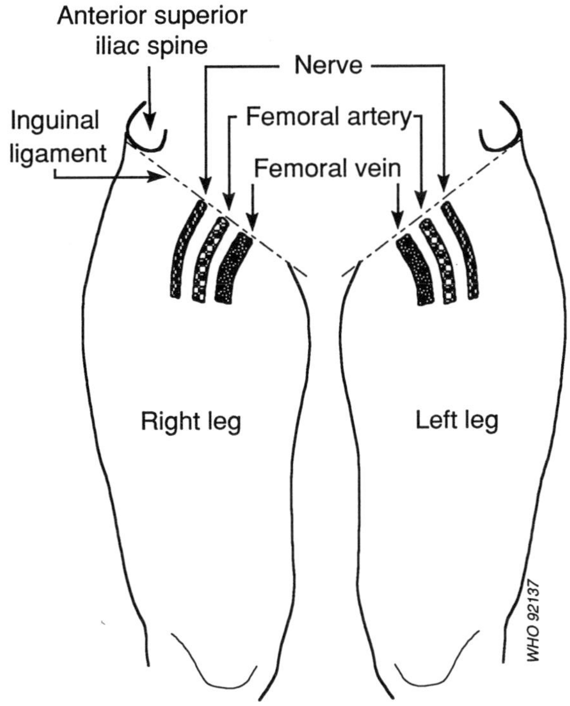

A. **The femoral vein is next to the femoral artery, on its medial side.**

B. **Locate the pulsation of the femoral artery with the fingers of one hand, and insert the needle vertically just medial to that location with the other hand. When blood fills the needle opening it is correctly positioned and the IV tubing can be connected. The needle must be held firmly in place while the IV infusion is running.**

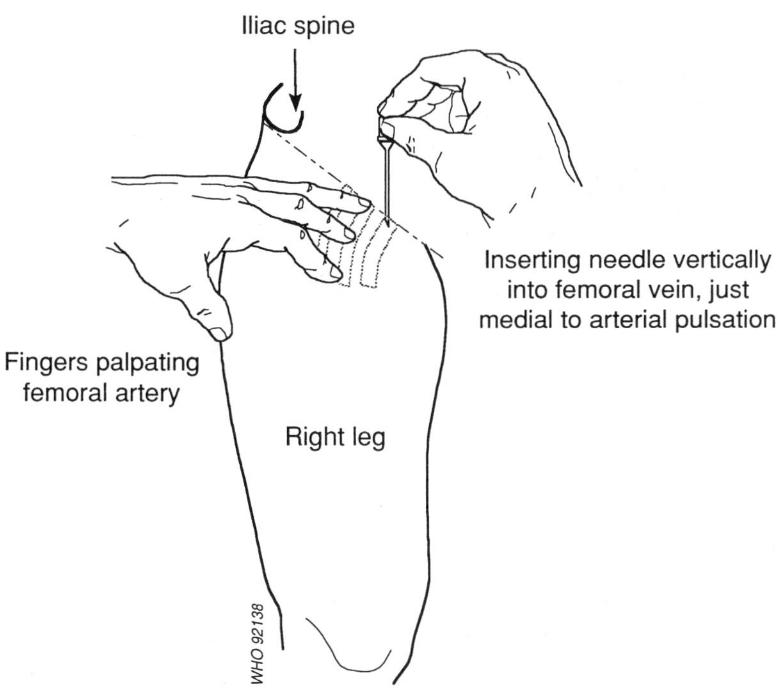

ANNEX 5

Nasogastric rehydration

1. Use a clean rubber or plastic nasogastric (NG) tube, 2.0–2.7 mm in diameter for a child, 4.0–6.0 mm for an adult.

2. Place the patient on his or her back, with the head slightly raised. Older children and adults may prefer to sit up.

3. Measure the length of tube which must be swallowed by placing the tip just above the navel. Then stretch the tubing over the back of the ear and forward to the tip of the nose. Mark the tube with a piece of tape where it touches the end of the nose. This mark shows the length of tubing needed to reach from the tip of the nose to the stomach.

4. Moisten the tube with a water-soluble lubricant or plain water; do not use oil.

5. Pass the tube through the side of the nose with the largest opening, and gently advance it until the tip is in the back of the throat. Each time the patient swallows, advance the tube 3–5 cm; if the patient is awake, ask him or her to drink a little water.

6. If the patient chokes, coughs repeatedly, or has trouble breathing, the tube has probably passed into the trachea. Pull it back 2–4 cm until the coughing stops and the patient is comfortable, wait a minute, and then try again.

7. Advance the tube each time the patient swallows until the tape marker reaches the nose. If the patient remains comfortable and is not coughing, the tube should be in the stomach.

8. Look into the patient's mouth to be certain the tube is not coiled in the back of the throat. Confirm that the tube is in the stomach by attaching a syringe and withdrawing a little stomach fluid; or place a stethoscope just above the navel, inject air into the tube with an empty syringe and listen for the air entering the stomach.

9. Fasten the tube to the face with tape and attach IV tubing that is connected to a clean IV bottle containing ORS solution. Regulate the infusion to a rate of 20 ml/kg per hour, or less.

10. If an IV bottle is not available, a syringe (with the barrel removed) can be attached to the tube and used as a funnel. Hold the syringe above the patient's head and pour ORS solution into it at regular intervals.

Technique for nasogastric rehydration

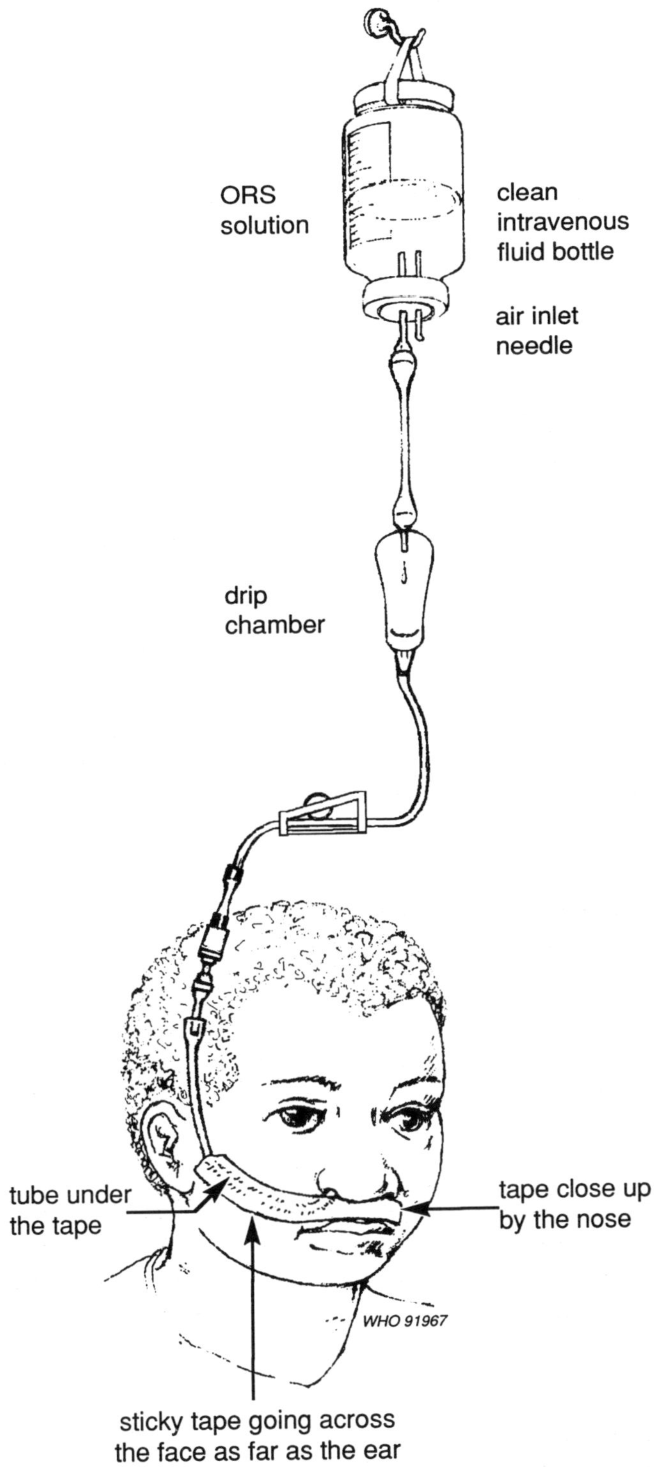

Source: King, M. et al. *Primary child care: a manual for health workers. Book One.* Oxford, Oxford University Press, 1978.

ANNEX 6

Antimicrobial agents used to treat specific causes of diarrhoea

Cause	Antimicrobial	Recommended dose		Estimated single dose (in tablets, capsules or ml of syrup), according to body weight in kg					
		Children	Adults	Children					Adults
				3–5 kg	6–9 kg	10–14 kg	15–19 kg	20–29 kg	
Cholera[1,2]	**Doxycycline[3]**								
	Tablet or capsule, 300 mg	Not suitable for children below 12 years	300 mg once	—	—	—	—	—	1
	Tetracycline								
	Tablet or capsule, 250 mg	12.5 mg/kg 4 times a day for 3 days	500 mg 4 times a day for 3 days	—	1/2 tablet	1	1	2	2
	Trimethoprim (TMP)–sulfamethoxazole (SMX)[4]								
	Adult tablet, TMP 80 mg and SMX 400 mg	TMP 5 mg/kg and SMX 25 mg/kg twice a day for 3 days	TMP 160 mg and SMX 800 mg twice a day for 3 days	1/4	1/2	1	1	2	2
	Paediatric tablet, TMP 20 mg and SMX 100 mg	TMP 5 mg/kg and SMX 25 mg/kg twice a day for 3 days	—	1	2	3	4	6	—

	Syrup, TMP 40 mg and SMX 200 mg in 5 ml	TMP 5 mg/kg and SMX 25 mg/kg twice a day for 3 days	—	2.5	5	7.5	10	15	—
	Furazolidone[5,6]								
	Tablet, 100 mg	1.25 mg/kg 4 times a day for 3 days	100 mg 4 times a day for 3 days	—	—	1/4	1/4	1/2	1
Dysentery[1,7]	**Trimethoprim (TMP)– sulfamethoxazole (SMX)**								
	Adult tablet, TMP 80 mg and SMX 400 mg	TMP 5 mg/kg and SMX 25 mg/kg twice a day for 5 days	TMP 160 mg and SMX 800 mg twice a day for 5 days	1/4	1/2	1	1	2	2
	Paediatric tablet, TMP 20 mg and SMX 100 mg	TMP 5 mg/kg and SMX 25 mg/kg twice a day for 5 days	—	1	2	3	4	6	—
	Syrup, TMP 40 mg and SMX 200 mg in 5 ml	TMP 5 mg/kg and SMX 25 mg/kg twice a day for 5 days	—	2.5	5	7.5	10	15	—
	Nalidixic acid								
	Tablet, 250 mg	15 mg/kg 4 times a day for 5 days	1 g 4 times a day for 5 days	1/4	1/2	1	1	2	4
	Ampicillin								
	Tablet or capsule, 250 mg	25 mg/kg 4 times a day for 5 days	1 g 4 times a day for 5 days	1/2 tablet	1	1	2	3	4

Annex 6 (*continued*)

Cause	**Antimicrobial**	**Recommended dose**		**Estimated single dose (in tablets, capsules or ml of syrup), according to body weight in kg**					
		Children	**Adults**	**Children**					**Adults**
				3–5 kg	**6–9 kg**	**10–14 kg**	**15–19 kg**	**20–29 kg**	
Amoebic dysentery[8]	**Metronidazole**								
	Tablet, 250 mg	10 mg/kg 3 times a day for 5 days (10 days for severe disease)	750 mg 3 times a day for 5 days (10 days for severe disease)	1/4	1/2	1/2	1	1	3
Giardiasis[9]	**Metronidazole**[10]								
	Tablet, 250 mg	5 mg/kg 3 times a day for 5 days	250 mg 3 times a day for 5 days	—	1/4	1/4	1/2	1/2	1

1 Selection of an antimicrobial should be based on sensitivity patterns of strains of *Vibrio cholerae* O1 and *Shigella* isolated in the area.

2 Antimicrobials are recommended for patients older than 2 years with suspected cholera and severe dehydration.

3 Doxycycline is the antimicrobial of choice for adults because only one dose is required. For treatment of pregnant women, see below.

4 Trimethoprim–sulfamethoxazole (also named co-trimoxazole) is the antimicrobial of choice for children. Tetracycline is equally effective; however, in some countries it is not recommended for paediatric use.

5 Furazolidone is the antimicrobial of choice for pregnant women.

6 Other choices include erythromycin and chloramphenicol.

7 *Shigella* is the most important cause of dysentery in young children. An antimicrobial to which most *Shigella* in the area are sensitive should be selected. If the stool is still bloody after two days, the antimicrobial should be stopped and a different one used.

8 Amoebiasis is an unusual cause of dysentery in young children. Metronidazole should be given only when trophozoites of *Entamoeba histolytica* containing red blood cells are seen in the faeces or when bloody stools persist after consecutive treatment with two antimicrobials (each given for two days) that are usually effective for *Shigella* in the area.

9 Treatment for giardiasis should be given only when diarrhoea is persistent (lasting at least 14 days) and cysts or trophozoites of *Giardia* are seen in the faeces or small bowel fluid.

10 Tinidazole and ornidazole are also effective. Tinidazole should be given in a single dose of 50 mg/kg orally (maximum dose 2 g). Ornidazole should be used in accordance with the manufacturer's recommendations.

Answers to exercises

Unit 1

1. A, B, C, D

2. E — Mohan has persistent diarrhoea, i.e. diarrhoea that begins acutely and lasts at least 14 days. The term chronic diarrhoea should not be used in this case; it refers to diarrhoea of long duration that is due to a noninfectious cause.

3. Viruses – rotavirus; bacteria – enterotoxigenic *Escherichia coli, Shigella, Campylobacter jejuni*; protozoa – *Cryptosporidium*.

4. A — The answer is 0%. The features of acute watery diarrhoea are not specific. It is not possible to determine *with certainty* the etiology of an episode of watery diarrhoea on the basis of the clinical features of the illness.

5. A, D — Antimicrobials are indicated only for dysentery (in which case treatment for shigellosis should be given) or for suspected cholera. Diarrhoea of longer than usual duration, diarrhoea with fever, and diarrhoea following exposure to animals do not benefit from antimicrobials.

6. D — Enterotoxigenic *Escherichia coli* (ETEC) is the most frequent cause of acute diarrhoea among cases detected in community surveys. None of the other agents listed are important causes of acute diarrhoea or dysentery in young children.

7. A, C, E — Some other protective behaviours are the use of a cup rather than a bottle to give milk formula, the use of clean drinking-water, cooking weaning foods well, thoroughly reheating any foods that are not eaten immediately after being cooked, and safe disposal of infant, adult, and animal faeces.

Unit 2

1. A–O
   B–S
   C–O
   D–S
   E–O

2. A, C, D, E

3. E — Hypovolaemia causes shock and cardiovascular collapse. This is the cause of death from severe dehydration due to diarrhoea.

4. A, C

5. A, B, E — Patients with paralytic ileus should not be given ORT; this will only make abdominal distension more severe. Patients with severe dehydration require very rapid replacement of water and salt to restore the blood volume and prevent death. ORT is not sufficiently rapid. Such patients need intravenous fluid replacement, if it is available.

6. B, E — The child would probably develop hypernatraemia because of the high concentrations of salt and glucose in the solution. Extreme thirst is a sign of hypernatraemia.

7. A, B, D — Soft drinks and commercial fruit drinks are often hyperosmolar owing to their high sugar content. Such fluids can cause osmotic diarrhoea and hypernatraemic dehydration. They also contain very little sodium to replace what has been lost.

Unit 3

1. B, C, E

2. C — The signs are those of *some dehydration.*

3. C — The signs of *some dehydration* are: irritable, fussy behaviour; taking water eagerly from a cup; and some decrease in skin turgor. These are all key signs and are sufficient to make the diagnosis of some dehydration. The treatment should follow Treatment Plan B.

4. B, D, E — Bantu has only one of the signs in Column B (irritable, restless behaviour); the rest are in Column A. Therefore, he has *no signs of dehydration.* As the stool contains blood he should be treated for dysentery. Because he has fever, a search should be made for evidence of an infection outside the intestinal tract. Pneumonia is an important possibility, especially if he is coughing and breathing rapidly.

5. A, B, C, D, E

Unit 4

1. A, B, C, D

2. A, B, D — Commercial fruit drinks and soft drinks are often hyperosmolar owing to their high sugar content. They also contain little or no sodium. If given to replace stool losses they could worsen the situation by causing osmotic diarrhoea and hypernatraemic dehydration.

3. A, B, C, D

4. A, C, D — Antimicrobials are not helpful in most episodes of acute diarrhoea. They should be used only for cases of dysentery and cases of suspected cholera with severe dehydration.

5. D — All of the described methods are helpful, but the *most* effective is letting the mother practise ORT under the supervision of a health worker.

Unit 5

1. B

2. B, D

3. B, C, D

4. B

5. B, C, D

6. A, D

7. A — Ria has severe dehydration.
   B — She requires 100 ml/kg, for a total of 600 ml.
   C — The fluid should be given intravenously.
   D — She should receive 30 ml/kg in the first hour, and 70 ml/kg in the next 5 hours.
   E — Codeine, possibly combined with a potassium deficit.

8. A — Hawa has severe dehydration, possibly caused by cholera.
   B — Normal saline solution (9 g NaCl/l), half-strength Darrow's solution with dextrose (25 g/l or 50 g/l) or half-normal saline with dextrose (50 g/l or 100 g/l).
   C — Hawa should receive an oral antimicrobial for cholera, usually tetracycline or doxycycline, after rehydration is complete and vomiting has stopped.
   D — Give Hawa small amounts of ORS solution as soon as she is able to drink; this should be possible after 1–2 hours of rehydration therapy.

9. A	Ali has some dehydration.
B	Treatment Plan B.
C	Ali should receive 200–400 ml of ORS solution during the first 4 hours.
D	The mother should resume breast-feeding at once and should continue to breast-feed during ORT.
E	Treatment Plan A should be used.

Unit 6

1. C, D, E	Absence of fever is not unusual in children with shigellosis or dysentery caused by other bacteria, especially when disease is severe. Even in this situation, amoebiasis is very unusual.
2. C, E	
3. D	
4. B	Answer D would be correct only if reliable laboratory facilities were readily available, which is not usually the case.
5. A, B, C, D, E	The reason Chinta should return for follow-up is that she had dysentery and was dehydrated when first seen.

Unit 7

1. E	A–D also occur but only contribute to weight loss if food intake is decreased. When enough food is given, weight loss is prevented.
2. A, B	
3. A, B, C, E	To avoid weight loss, Yunus should be given a nutrient-rich diet throughout the episode of diarrhoea.
4. A, C	
5. A, D, E	
6. Part 1–B	Demonstrating a close association between diarrhoea and milk feeds is the most important. Testing the stool for pH and reducing substances is only helpful to confirm the diagnosis when it is clear that milk makes the diarrhoea worse.
Part 2–B, C, D	

Unit 8

1. B, C, D

2. C — Healthy, breast-fed infants below 4 months of age do not require any other food or fluids. Giving these increases the risk of diarrhoea.

3. A, B, C, D, E

4. B, D

5. A, C, D